Joslin Diabetes Manual

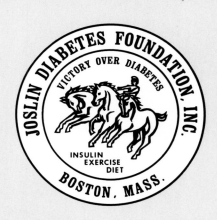
JOSLIN DIABETES FOUNDATION, INC.

VICTORY OVER DIABETES

INSULIN
EXERCISE
DIET

BOSTON, MASS.

Joslin
Diabetes
Manual

*by Physicians of the Joslin Clinic Division
of the Joslin Diabetes Foundation, Inc.*

Edited by LEO P. KRALL, M.D.

*Director, Education Division, Joslin Diabetes Foundation;
Lecturer in Medicine, Harvard Medical School, Boston,
Mass.; Editor-in-Chief,* Diabetes Forecast, *American Diabetes
Association, New York; Vice-President of the International
Diabetes Federation, London.*

ELEVENTH EDITION

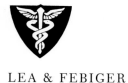

LEA & FEBIGER   'PHILADELPHIA

First Edition, 1918
Second Edition, 1919
Third Edition, 1924
Fourth Edition, 1929
Fifth Edition, 1934
Sixth Edition, 1937
Seventh Edition, 1941
Eighth Edition, 1948
Ninth Edition, 1953
Tenth Edition, 1959

Library of Congress Cataloging in Publication Data

Main entry under title:

Joslin diabetes manual.

   Completely rewritten, rev., and modernized ed.
of A diabetic manual for the mutual use of doctor
and patient, by E. P. Joslin.
   Includes bibliographical references and index.
   1. Diabetes.   I. Krall, Leo P.   II. Joslin,
Elliott Proctor, 1869–1962. A diabetic manual for
the mutual use of doctor and patient.   III. Joslin
Diabetes Foundation. [DNLM: 1. Diabetes
mellitus—Popular works. WK850 J84j]
RC660.J58   1978   616.4′62   77-29115
ISBN 0-8121-0607-5

Published in Great Britain by Henry Kimpton Publishers, London
PRINTED IN THE UNITED STATES OF AMERICA
Print Number 10   9   8   7   6   5   4   3   2

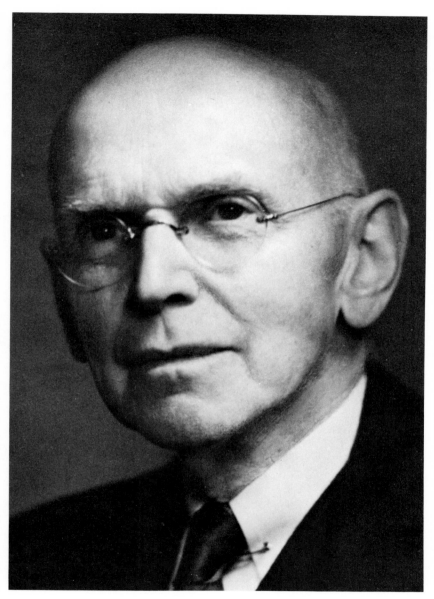

ELLIOTT P. JOSLIN, M.D.
1869-1962

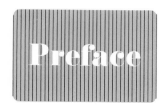

Preface

You may be reading the half-millionth copy of this Manual. That is a tribute to the late Elliott P. Joslin, who understood the importance of patient education in the treatment of diabetes mellitus and who wrote the first edition in 1918. Since Dr. Joslin's death in 1962, there have been no further editions, and worn, tattered copies of the tenth edition are still in use in many parts of the world.

It would be impossible to attempt to follow in the footsteps of the original teacher. Changes have taken place in medicine much as they have in many other areas. When Dr. Joslin started his medical practice at the beginning of the century, not much was known about diabetes; certainly, there were no teaching centers until many years later. Eventually, Dr. Joslin's practice evolved into the Joslin Clinic, and in 1968 the Clinic joined forces with the Diabetes Foundation to form the Joslin Diabetes Foundation. Now, many good facilities exist nationwide for the care and education of the diabetic patient, and this wide dispersion can only be considered a gain for our increasing population of diabetic persons. No single institution can claim a monopoly of knowledge regarding diabetes, and while philosophies of treatment among institutions may differ in degree of emphasis, the important point is that those who suffer from this disease are receiving better care every day.

The available information and experience regarding diabetes and other diseases have burgeoned to such a degree that the individual physician cannot serve his patients fully without help from other professionals. Thus, many individuals—phy-

sicians, nurses, dietitians, technicians, and social workers—
comprise the treatment and teaching team. Each is skilled in a
different discipline, but all are dedicated to the betterment of
the patient's life.

A book of this type represents a brew of the knowledge
distilled from the experience of many. We borrow from our
predecessors even as, hopefully, our achievements may be
helpful to the next generation. At best one compiles, evaluates,
edits, rewrites and focuses the ideas of many others. For example, nothing could be written for diabetics without consulting the many decades of clinical experience amassed by
Drs. Elliott P. Joslin, Howard F. Root and Alexander Marble. It
would be impossible to discuss diabetes in mothers and children without the guidance of Dr. Priscilla White's 50 years of
clinical practice. Dr. Allen P. Joslin, son of the founder, is
known to thousands of patients because of his warm concern.
He and the other Clinic physicians who care for more than
43,000 patients each year have likewise collaborated in the
writing of this manual. They are:

Lloyd M. Aiello, M.D.   Gisella G. Garan, M.D.
Donald M. Barnett, M.D.   H. Howard Goldstein, M.D.
Robert F. Bradley, M.D.   Charles A. Graham, M.D.
Edward J. Busick, Jr, M.D.   William B. Hadley, M.D.
A. Richard Christlieb, M.D.   John W. Hare, M.D.
Ramachandiran Cooppan, M.D. George P. Kozak, M.D.
John A. D'Elia, M.D.   Donna Younger, M.D.
B. Dan Ferguson, M.D.   Louis Vignati, M.D.
Thomas M. Flood, M.D.

Senior investigators of the Elliott P. Joslin Research Labor-
atory, directed by Dr. George F. Cahill, Jr., have also made
critical and informative changes in the text. These include
Drs. Arthur A. Like, Aldo A. Rossini, Neil B. Ruderman and
J. Stuart Soeldner. The bulk of teaching at the Joslin Diabetes
Foundation is now done by Miss Denise Stevens, M.A.T., and
the teaching nurses, along with the New England Deaconess
Hospital and Clinic nurses and dietitians and aides; I thank
them for their contributions. Finally, I wish to acknowledge
Diane Zaromskis and Dr. Aldo Rossini who, in addition to
myself, provided illustrations for this Manual.

Never has there been so much information available about diabetes as now. Many of the older concepts have changed, but we now have cogent reasons to support some long-held beliefs which, although correct, had been previously unproven. In addition to imparting the basic knowledge that should enable diabetics to survive better, we have made a conscious effort in writing this Manual to translate information into the modern idiom using contemporary terms.

With deep respect for the past and a keen eye on the future, we must always remember that those who need help are here, now!

LEO P. KRALL, M.D.

Boston, Massachusetts

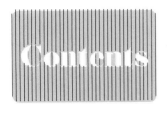

Contents

Appendices 280

Joslin
Diabetes
Manual

What is Diabetes?

Why are you reading this book? Why are you interested in diabetes? Do you have it? A child, a parent, a relative, a friend of yours? There may be many good reasons for learning about diabetes, but one of the best reasons is the fact that knowledge and understanding can help you or someone else live better and longer as well as freer from complications. Simple survival is not enough. To cope with the diabetic life depends largely on how much you know.

If you have diabetes, you are one of an increasing number of persons so afflicted. The National Commission on Diabetes, which consists of leaders in diabetes care, research and administration, reported to Congress in late 1975 that "diabetes is a major health problem directly affecting as many as 10 million Americans. . . . Between 1965 and 1973 the prevalence of diabetes increased by more than 50% in the United States. Diabetes now affects 5% of the population. In 1974 more than 600,000 new cases of diabetes were diagnosed and the incidence of diabetes appears to be increasing by 6% per year. At this rate, the number of those with diabetes will double every 15 years." So you are not alone!

However, the Commission also points out that people faced with a lifelong problem like diabetes "are understandably plagued by fear and in need of education and counseling." Diabetes needs daily attention. The report also recommends that the families of diabetics should learn about the necessary care and treatment in order to understand how to help and how to live with a person who has diabetes.

As discussed later in this book, evidence increasingly shows that emphasizing good care and exerting a sustained effort to achieve a physiology that is as normal as possible may not only make the course of the condition smoother, but also may prevent complications. This means that acquiring knowledge leading to better care is not a luxury, but a necessity.

Although a physician can offer guidance during a limited number of office or hospital visits yearly, the person with diabetes must live with it 365 days a year and be prepared to cope constantly with the problems of everyday life. Knowledge and understanding are not a part of treatment; they *are* treatment.

definition of diabetes

By definition, diabetes is a state caused by insufficient available insulin. For about 75 years it was thought that diabetes was a simple condition, involving only an insufficient amount of insulin, and that if this insulin defect were corrected, diabetes would be cured. Although this may still be true in general, enough has been learned to suggest that the condition is indeed much more complex.

Antagonists that render insulin less effective, interference by other hormones, and even an inability of some cell receptors to accept the insulin effect may also be a part of the problem, as well as not enough insulin. Even the wonderful discovery of insulin in 1921, while saving countless lives and permitting diabetics to live, has not always prevented the occurrence of complications in diabetics. This may be due to our present methods of delivery and timing of insulin. The treatment as often practiced is not always physiological; therefore, it does not offer optimal protection. This does not mean that we know little about diabetes; it simply suggests that diabetes may be related to other problems besides the inability of the pancreas to make enough insulin. The problem is similar to having a jigsaw puzzle for which many pieces are present but more pieces must be found to create a complete, clear picture of diabetes. Again, this is not to say that little is known about diabetes—*more* is known than ever before.

If one were to ask a group of various scientists about what diabetes means to them, differences of opinion would evolve, depending on the training of the specialist. For instance, the pathologist would state that diabetes is a disease that affects all the tissues of the body but in particular the small blood vessels of the kidney, eye and even the nervous system. The physiologist might state that certain materials that alter the functions of different organs are deposited in diabetes. On the other hand, a biochemist might state that it is a disease in which blood sugar levels are elevated, characterized not only by insulin deficiency but by changes in certain hormones, enzymes and other body substances. An expert in epidemiology might emphasize the fact that diabetes affects 5% of the American population and that this number is increasing. The geneticist would point to the strong hereditary predisposition of individuals for diabetes. The cardiologist would note that diabetes is a leading cause of heart disease in the United States, and the eye specialist would state that diabetes is a leading cause of decreased vision and blindness.

The physician who takes care of diabetics must be an all-purpose person who understands internal medicine, biochemistry, cardiology, ophthalmology, dermatology, neurology, urology, pediatrics and many other areas of medicine, as well as human psychology. He must indeed be a medical "man for all seasons." The physician of today is better prepared to deal with all the problems of diabetes than ever before.

The fact that we do not know *everything* about diabetes should not be discouraging, because the increasing number of clinical and research findings of the past dozen years have given us not only new answers, but fresh insight about more important answers soon to come. Diabetes can be diagnosed in most cases, and it can be adequately treated, which is not true of many other chronic conditions.

historical interest

The first actual description of diabetes dates back some 1500 years before Christ. In the centuries near the beginning of Christianity, the appearance of diabetes in succeeding generations was described. The famous works of Susruta (400 B.C.), of India, and his disciple, Charaka (6 A.D.), noted many of the symptoms and even the types of diabetes. Aretaeus (2 A.D.) used the general term "diabetes," which is an Ionic Greek word meaning "to run through a siphon." Although the Indian name for diabetes, "Madhumeha" or "honey-urine," was used in the sixth century A.D., the Latin word "mellitus" (honey) was applied much later. Even in this early period of history, observers noted that heredity was important, because various members of the same family were afflicted with the "sweet-water disease." During this period of history, another type of diabetes was recorded, maturity-onset diabetes, in which, in addition to the usual symptoms, the patient was both obese and without energy. The other type of diabetes (with onset in youth) was described as "melting down the flesh" and producing a sweet urine. Historical descriptions of the disease by Thomas Wills, Dodson and Claude Bernard all gave significance to the condition and the recognition of complications. The descriptions of diabetes now show similar findings.

In the nineteenth century, Brockman, in his study of fish, and later Langerhans, in his study of humans, described clusters of cells present in the pancreas (sweet bread) as little islands in a sea of pancreatic tissue. These islets make up a small 1% of the total pancreas. Two German scientists, von Mering and Minkowski, noted in 1889 that if the pancreas were removed, the animal developed diabetes. Later scientists discovered that even if the pancreas were destroyed, the animals did not become diabetic if the islets were preserved. The studies of Opie in the United States confirmed the fact that the small islets were damaged in humans with diabetes. Using this preliminary information available in 1921, plus the earlier works contributed by other scientists around the world, Banting and Best in Ontario, Canada (*Fig. 1*), began an important and historical research project. When they obtained the minced and purified islet tissues from animals and injected the material into an animal with diabetes, they found that the blood sugar levels fell. This was an important event for the many thousands of diabetics throughout the world and signaled a whole new era in the treatment of diabetes. At one stroke, life was substituted for death for the multitudes of people with diabetes!

Although this discovery was believed to be the solution to the problems of diabetes, it eventually became apparent that the simple intermittent administration of insulin was not sufficient to alter the basic diabetes state in many patients. Although many diabetics seem to escape most or all complications, others are less fortunate. This raises many questions. Are patients treated with insulin (or insulin-producing agents) early enough or constantly enough? Does something destroy or

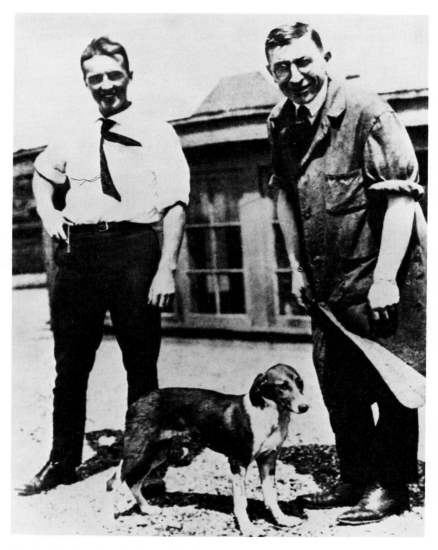

FIG. 1. Charles Best (left) and Dr. Frederick Banting, with the first dog treated successfully with insulin in 1921. At that time Charles Best was a graduate student, involved with both departments of biology and physiology at the University of Toronto. Dr. Banting was a surgeon. (Courtesy of Charles Best and Eli Lilly Co.)

inhibit the action of insulin? Does vascular damage occur regardless of insulin therapy? Answers to these questions are gradually forthcoming. As suggested earlier, today's treatment methods may have to be revised to correspond more closely to the production and release of insulin in the nondiabetic individual.

the function of the pancreas

The pancreas is situated below and behind the stomach (*Fig. 2*). The gland weighs about a half pound, and within the pancreas, especially in the tail, are very small pieces of tissue called islets of Langerhans. These contain beta cells (described in 1869), which secrete insulin. Aside from the manufacture, storage and release of insulin, the pancreas has several important functions. One is the production of certain enzymes important for the conversion of various foods in the diet. When proteins, starches, or even more complicated foods are eaten, the pancreas secretes and releases through a duct into the intestines certain enzymes that digest this large, bulky food

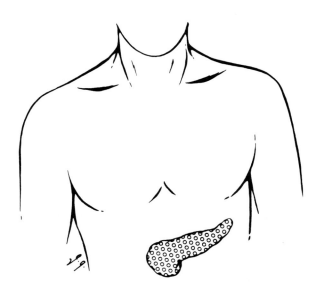

FIG. 2. The relative position of the pancreas, which lies below and behind the stomach.

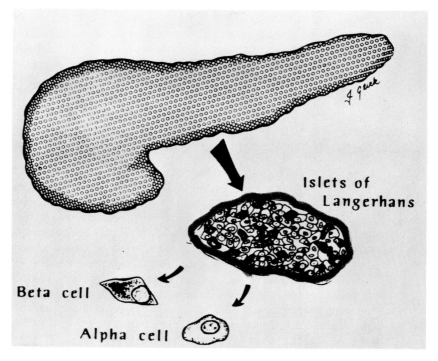

FIG. 3. Diagram showing the relative density of the islets of Langerhans in the pancreas. One of the dots is enlarged to show the actual position of the alpha (glucagon-secreting) and beta (insulin-secreting) cells in the islets of Langerhans.

into simpler substances, which can be absorbed into the bloodstream and transported throughout the body for direct use or storage.

Another major function of the pancreas is the production and release of glucagon by the alpha cells (*Fig. 3*). The absorption of protein from the diet stimulates the release of glucagon. A main function of glucagon is to raise the blood glucose level; thus one might say that glucagon has an anti-insulin function. The balance in the insulin-glucagon relationship seems to be important in influencing the normal blood glucose range.

The pancreas also contains numerous delta cells, whose function has recently been described as probably producing somatostatin, which mediates between glucagon and insulin.

> ## THE WONDERFUL WORLD OF BETA CELLS!
>
> Each normal pancreas has about 100,000 islets of Langerhans, and each islet contains between 80 and 100 beta cells. These cells are capable of measuring the blood glucose level every 10 seconds to within a range of 2 mg. per cent. Within 60 to 90 seconds, the beta cells can organize themselves to deliver any amount of insulin necessary.

the production of insulin

The first product made by the beta cells in the islets is called *proinsulin*, which is a chain of 81 amino acids (basic proteins). This chain is transferred to an area of the cell called the Golgi apparatus. Here the proinsulin is broken down into two units. Fifty-one of the amino acids remain, and this chain is now *insulin*. The remaining 30 amino acids are known as C- (or connecting) peptide. Both these units are then stored in tiny storage droplets to be released when necessary in response to stimulation. The C-peptide has no known effect but is released into the circulation with the insulin molecule, much like a first-stage rocket shell being released and discarded when a spaceship goes into orbit (*Fig. 4*). The C-peptide, therefore, may be useful as a "marker" by which technicians can determine the degree of function of the beta cells.

The beta cell, when stimulated by glucose as well as other foods in the diet, releases insulin in two stages. The first stage involves release of the insulin already stored within the beta cells. The second stage is much more complicated. With the increase in the level of glucose in the blood, a signal is sent to the nucleus (or "brain") of the beta cell, which relays this information to the production area, and more insulin is produced. A similar situation might be drawn: a factory manager sends a message to his production department to increase their output when he learns that more of his product is needed. The boss, in fact, might send his son, who would go to the production manager. The son gives the foreman the production plans and goals (the cellular process of "transcription of information" is known as the role of messenger RNA). Once the plans

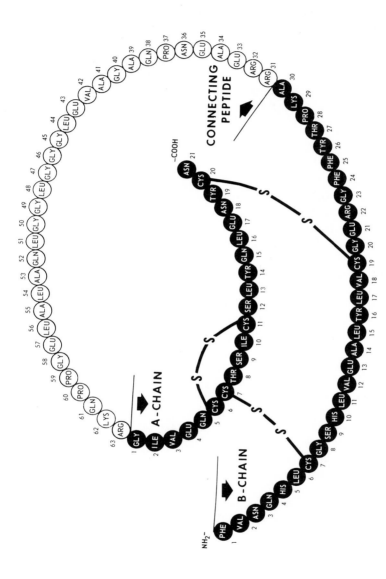

FIG. 4. Insulin and proinsulin. As discussed in the text, the entire structure is proinsulin, which precedes insulin. Insulin (the dark lower portion) is released from the parent structure. When discarded, the lighter upper portion is known as "C-peptide." The letters and numbers for each circle identify the individual amino acids (protein) that make up these substances. The sequence of the amino acids is specific for each species. The animal whose amino acid sequence for insulin is closest to man's is the pig. (Courtesy of Eli Lilly Co.)

are determined, the raw materials and equipment are arranged to put the product together. In the actual cell, the messenger RNA sets up the tools and pattern whereby the raw materials are used to assemble the insulin molecule.

When a person eats bread, for example, it is broken down (digested) and absorbed chiefly as sugar into the bloodstream, where the increased blood sugar level stimulates the release of insulin. However, insulin formation starts even before the blood sugar (glucose) level becomes elevated. As food enters the digestive tract, certain hormones are released, and these stimulate the release of insulin from the beta cells. Further manufacture and release of insulin depend on the amount and type of food eaten. Carbohydrates (sugars and starches) are potent insulin-release stimulators. The increasing blood sugar level stimulates more insulin formation and release in a sustained flow.

In the nondiabetic, it is almost impossible to raise the blood glucose level significantly, since the amount of available insulin is almost inexhaustible—not too much and not too little, just precisely the correct amount. In fact, if a person were to get a slow infusion of 5% glucose in a vein of one arm, the levels of glucose in blood from a vein in the other arm would most often be normal. The person without diabetes can manufacture and release 40 to 50 units of insulin daily, and have several hundred units available in pancreatic storage for release as needed. A truly remarkable mechanism!

the function of insulin

Once the insulin is in the circulation, it performs definite and vital roles. In simple terms, insulin is the main messenger that gives the body signals that control the storage and mobilization of fuels. To simplify this further and to show the relationship between insulin and body fuel, the body may be described as a machine. This analogy will also explain what happens and what symptoms occur in the state of diabetes.

How the Diabetes Machine Works.   A machine, for instance, a motorcycle, functions by allowing a combustible material to be ignited by a spark (*Fig.* 5), producing an explosion that provides a source of energy to move a piston. Motion

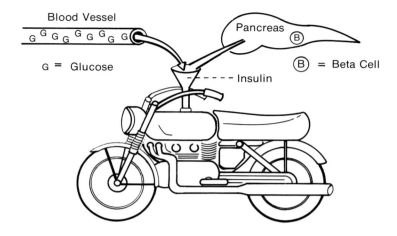

Blood Vessel

G = Glucose

Pancreas

(B) = Beta Cell

Insulin

THE DIABETES MACHINE

FIG. 5. The body can be compared to a motorcycle. Instead of gasoline, the body uses fuels such as glucose to provide the energy to make it run. Insulin acts like a funnel that aids the distribution of fuel into the body cells, where energy is produced. (Adapted from Rossini, A.: The great diabetes machine. Diabetes Forecast, 29:22, 1976.)

is transmitted to the wheels by certain gears and the result is movement of the motorcycle. The faster the pickup in speed of the machine, the greater the use of fuel and the more combustion, the swifter is the motion of the motorcycle. The body works on the same principle, using fuels that can be either glucose, proteins (amino acids) or fats (fatty acids). These can be changed inside the machine through a complicated combustion system known to scientists as the "Krebs cycle." This forms an energy substance called ATP (adenosine triphosphate). This ATP provides the energy necessary for function of our machine in a normal living state. It is used to keep the heart, the brain, the liver and the kidney functioning, as well as to provide energy for such demanding activities as walking or running. The end products of fuel combustion, in both motorcycle and body, are carbon dioxide, water and energy. The machine disposes of these products by way of the tail pipe, while in the body they escape through the lungs and kidney.

In the case of the motorcycle, an attendant in a gas station provides the fuel needed for the machine through a hose and nozzle. In the body, the fuels enter from the stomach and intestines into the circulation, and in the presence of insulin, the fuels are able to enter the body cells where they are used. Thus, the body machine requires insulin as a means for the fuel to enter into the machine for the production of energy (*Fig.* 6).

Fuel for the Machine. Many types of fuels can be used for the motorcycle besides gasoline. For example, kerosene, methyl alcohol (methanol) or oils can be used when nothing else is available. The body uses three types of fuel: carbohydrates, protein and fat.

CARBOHYDRATES. Carbohydrate is readily found in the usual diet (fruits, vegetables, cakes, bread and potatoes). These foods in the body are easily changed into simple small sugars, mainly glucose. This happens in the intestine and liver with the help of various enzyme reactions. The final result is glu-

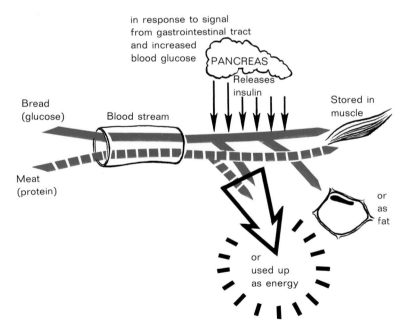

FIG. 6. Mechanism of insulin release, which enables the food fuels to be used for the production of energy or stored for future use.

cose, which goes into the circulation (*Fig. 7*). These glucose molecules stimulate the beta cells in the pancreas to release insulin, which permits the fuel (glucose) to enter the machine (cell). The body can store much of the fuel if excess amounts are taken in and not used. Through the effect of insulin, glucose can be converted in the liver into animal "starch" or glycogen, which can be stored in the liver and the skeletal muscles. Extra quantities of unused glucose are also changed into fats, which can be retained in storage depots in adipose tissue. These reserves of fuels can be reconverted into glucose for quick energy in times of need. If the blood sugar level falls, the fuels that are stored in the form of glycogen or fats are released back into the circulation to produce the fuel to keep the machine running. This rapid availability of glucose occurs when there is a fuel shortage (low blood sugar). Even the small amount of glucose produced will then stimulate enough release of fuels in the body. Thus, a fine balance exists between insulin levels and the stored fuels. It is important to remember that ingestion of too much carbohydrate, glucose or, for that matter, any fuel can produce an increase in fat, which then continues to develop into a state known as obesity. The obese person has large storage cells, all excessively filled with fat.

PROTEIN.   Protein is available from the daily diet (meat, cheese, fish). When such foods enter the intestines, enzymes break them down into smaller compounds called amino acids. Once they enter the circulation, amino acids also may stimulate insulin release from the beta cell. The fate of these amino acids is much like that of carbohydrate; they are used as fuel when insulin is present (*Fig. 8*). They are also used to supply building blocks for muscle protein as well as the production of enzymes. The amino acids can likewise be converted to glucose in the liver. The ability of the liver to trap these amino acids and convert them to glucose is helped by the other pancreatic hormone, glucagon. The fate of this glucose is similar to that of excess glucose mentioned previously. It can be converted to glycogen or fat for storage purposes.

FAT.   The third and final fuel for the human metabolic machine is fat, as found in oils from corn, peanuts and olives, as well as fat in meat, fowl, butter and other dairy products such as milk, cream and cheese. These foods are digested and

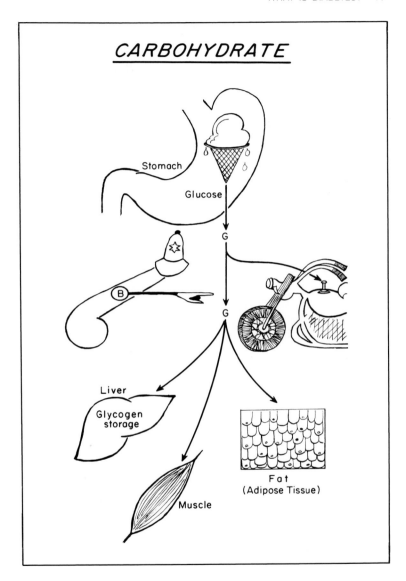

FIG. 7. Carbohydrate is the most readily usable fuel for the body. It is found in sugars and starches; around the world, it is the most available type of food. In this example, ice cream has been eaten and broken down into glucose. Insulin, like a traffic policeman (B), permits the fuel to enter the machine (body cells), where it can be used at once or stored in the liver, muscles, or fat for future use. (From Rossini, A.: The great diabetes machine. Diabetes Forecast, 29:22, 1976.)

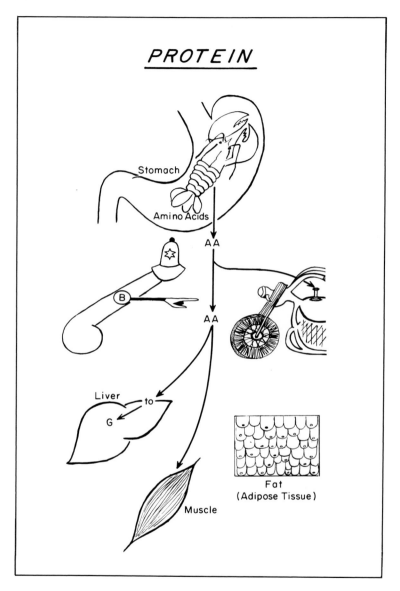

FIG. 8. Protein is an important type of fuel, sources of which include meat, seafood, and dairy products. Protein is broken down into smaller particles called amino acids; insulin has to be present before amino acids can be used for energy by the body. This fuel is used more slowly than glucose. (From Rossini, A.: The great diabetes machine. Diabetes Forecast, 29:22, 1976.)

absorbed into the bloodstream where they are converted into
fatty acids for use in the body (*Fig. 9*). The excess fat in the
circulation, under the influence of insulin, can go directly into
fat cells and be stored as reserves that are available when fuels
are low, during sleep or after a prolonged period without food.
Fat, however, is never converted into glucose. It can either go
into the machine and be used as a fuel directly in the form of
fatty acids, or be stored as a potential fuel in the fat cells for
use at a later date.

How Diabetes Affects the Machine. As mentioned earlier,
diabetes is basically a deficiency of insulin (*Fig. 10*). When
insulin levels are low, major changes occur. The fuel cannot
enter the machine, and the body reacts in a manner similar to
a machine that is low on fuel, namely, it begins to function
poorly and sputter. In the human, the early symptoms of
diabetes may be tiredness, weakness, and an inability to produce enough energy to perform well. The normally active
young child may be chronically fatigued. When fuel cannot
enter the machine, the sensation of hunger appears and the
individual overeats (polyphagia). Since insulin levels are low
and no insulin is released into the circulation from stimulation by food, an accumulation of glucose and other fuels takes
place. The stored fuels in the form of glycogen, fat and amino
acids in the muscle protein are broken down and enter the
circulation to supply the needs of the body cells for nourishment. Thus, very high glucose and fat levels occur in the
circulation, but these fuels cannot be converted for use by the
hungry cell because of the lack of insulin. This overload of
unused glucose circulates through the kidney. Normally, the
kidney would retrieve the useful glucose, but in this instance,
so much extra glucose is available that it spills over into the
urine, like excessive water flowing over a dam. The usual
kidney threshold for glucose is between 160 and 180 mg. per
cent in the blood (*Fig. 11*). When the blood sugar level is
higher than this, glucose spills over into the urine, which is
excreted in copious amounts. The sugar in the urine is called
glycosuria, and the loss of large amounts of urine is known as
polyuria. This loss of large amounts of water stimulates an
effort to increase the amount of body water by increasing the
sensation of thirst (polydipsia). So the vicious cycle of untreated diabetes brings on the classic symptoms of tiredness,
weakness, loss of glucose and excessive water in the urine

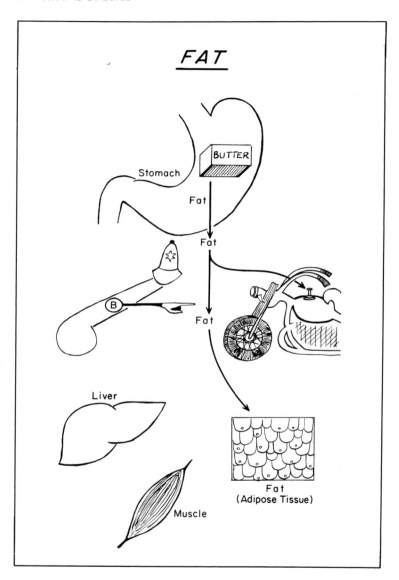

FIG. 9. Fat is the third type of fuel available to the body, although not as rapidly as glucose. Sources of fat include meat and dairy products and vegetable oils. As with other fuels, insulin must be present before fats can be taken into the machine (body cells); in this case, some fat is being stored in fat cells for future emergencies. If not used, it remains in storage. (Courtesy of A. Rossini)

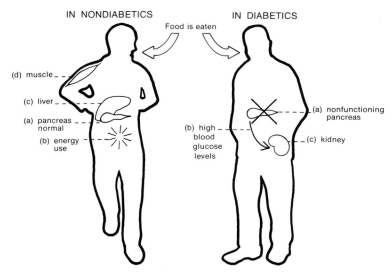

FIG. 10. In *nondiabetics,* the pancreas (a) releases enough insulin to enable the body to use food as energy (b) and to store excess nutrients in the liver and muscles (c,d). In *diabetics,* a nonfunctioning pancreas (a) results in an insulin shortage, so that food cannot be used for fuel. The blood levels of glucose are high (b), and glucose is lost through the kidney (c) into the urine.

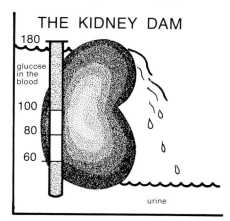

FIG. 11. The kidney dam. The figures 60 to 100 mg. per 100 ml. of blood show the normal fasting level of glucose in the blood. Ordinarily glucose does not appear in the urine until much higher levels are reached (ordinarily between 160 to 180 mg. per 100 ml. of blood or higher). In this respect, the kidney can be considered a dam. (Adapted from Rossini, A.: The great diabetes machine. Diabetes Forecast, 29:22, 1976.)

(polyuria), marked thirst (polydipsia) and hunger (polyphagia) and weight loss. Another result of diabetes may be the formation, from the excessive breakdown of stored fat, of materials known as ketone acids. These acids are produced by the liver when the fat released from the fat cell enters into the circulation with insufficient insulin to handle it. This may produce severe acidosis which, carried to extreme, can threaten life itself. Before the discovery of insulin, patients with severe acidosis often did not survive. Now, with the availability of injectable insulin, a patient can supplement his own deficient insulin by injecting insulin. The end result permits the fuels to enter the machine, thereby switching off the great loss of stored fuels. This, in turn, eliminates the symptoms of diabetes.

types of diabetes

As mentioned, diabetes occurs in two major forms: juvenile-onset and maturity-onset. Although the terms seem to imply that only young people have juvenile and older people maturity-type diabetes, this is not true. The major differences involve the type of onset and the character of the disease. In juvenile-onset diabetes, the symptoms usually occur rapidly and dramatically because the beta cells produce very little, if any, insulin. On the other hand, in maturity-onset diabetes, the symptoms may occur much more insidiously. Since the younger diabetic usually has no insulin, replacement by injection of insulin is necessary to control the diabetic state. The maturity-onset diabetic usually produces some insulin and has milder symptoms; often the diabetes can be controlled by dietary restrictions alone. In addition, the sulfonylurea compounds may aid by stimulating insulin release. Other oral hypoglycemic agents (biguanides), which function primarily by altering the machinery of the body through other routes, lower blood glucose levels. The typical maturity-onset diabetic is often obese and develops the disease after the age of 40. This group may include as many as 85% of all diabetics. The remaining 15% are those, usually under age 40 at onset and often thin, who ordinarily require injection of insulin in addition to diet regulation. It must be emphasized that the juvenile-onset type of diabetes occurs in a sizable number of older diabetics as well (perhaps 15 to 20%). The maturity-onset type may occur in a small number (perhaps 5%) of diabetics who are under the age of 20 years.

In normal persons, the body is able to produce just enough insulin to match the fuel supplied by eating. There is neither too much nor too little. If a person eats too much food beyond that which can be used as energy, he or she becomes obese by storing the extra calories. If this process continues, the insulin demands become greater. If the pancreas can produce enough insulin, the blood sugar levels may still remain normal. However, if the beta cell either is defective because of heredity or previous damage or if it simply becomes grossly overworked, the demand for insulin eventually exceeds the supply and the symptoms of diabetes occur. At times, obese persons seem to have insulin levels that are normal and possibly above normal, but still have a *relative* lack because their larger body mass requires more insulin. There is now reason to believe that fewer "receptor areas" exist on the cells themselves, so that the deficiency is compounded. Furthermore, the increased demand for more insulin means that eventually the *apparent* lack of enough insulin becomes *real*. The ideal treatment is to decrease the food intake through diet regulation. This permits better use of the available insulin and decreases the demand for the manufacture of more insulin. The reduced body mass also aids in balancing the metabolic cycle. On the other hand, if the adult with symptoms and findings of diabetes is not obese and does not have the ability to provide enough of his or her own insulin, other treatment measures must be taken.

COMMON SYMPTOMS OF DIABETES:

HUNGER (polyphagia)
THIRST (polydipsia)
FREQUENT URINATION (polyuria)
WEIGHT LOSS
TIREDNESS
SEVERE IRRITATION AND ITCHING (especially in the vaginal or rectal area, sometimes accompanied by FREQUENT INFECTIONS)

The DIAGNOSIS of diabetes mellitus must be confirmed by blood and urine glucose tests.

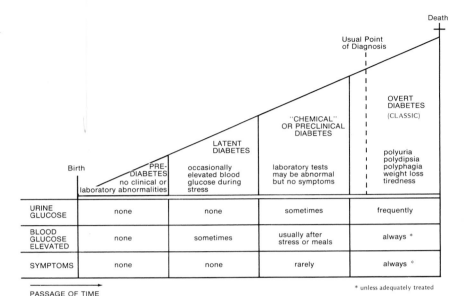

FIG. 12. The natural history of diabetes mellitus. Too often the diagnosis is made after the classic symptoms have been apparent for some time.

natural history of diabetes (*Fig. 12*)

Besides the two main types of diabetes, another classification divides diabetes into stages that are related to the passage of time, or possibly to the duration of the disease. These compartments are not air-tight, because while some persons progress steadily through the various stages, others become no worse, and indeed sometimes the situation appears to improve so that the subject reverts to a "milder" stage of diabetes.

PREDIABETES. This is a purely theoretical period; this classification usually is reserved for those individuals who have both parents with diabetes or who have an identical twin who has diabetes. Such a person not only has no signs or symptoms of diabetes, but actually has no abnormal blood or urine glucose tests even under provocation with glucose or cortisone. This person may never become diabetic, but is considered a "probable" diabetic, "diabetes-prone," or a "suspect."

LATENT DIABETES.   This term is applied to a person who has the elevated blood glucose levels of diabetes only in certain times of stress. For example, diabetic blood sugar levels may occur during pregnancy or during a severe infection. These symptoms often disappear when the pregnancy ends or after recovery from the infection.

CHEMICAL OR PRECLINICAL DIABETES (so called because no symptoms are present).   With this type of diabetes, a person, when not eating, has sufficient insulin to maintain normal levels of blood sugars (normal fasting blood sugar). However, after eating or taking glucose, the blood glucose levels are abnormally high and glucose may appear in the urine. These persons generally produce some but not enough insulin. The course of the disease frequently becomes more severe if the factors influencing diabetes are not changed. Such persons may become the diabetics of the future.

OVERT DIABETES.   This person has elevated blood sugar levels almost all of the time. The category includes those classic types of diabetes described previously. Unfortunately, diabetes in the adult is often not diagnosed until this stage is reached, although evidence suggests that vigorous treatment early can often influence the course for the better.

the causes of diabetes

Differentiating absolutely between factors that cause diabetes and those that represent the effects of diabetes is often diffi-cult. We know that the blood sugar level is elevated, but the cause of this elevated level is not certain aside from the fact that the amount of insulin is insufficient. Is this due to defec-tive beta cells, to an excess of some hormone in the circulation or to something that causes insulin to be ineffective? A sum-mary of some of the factors that might help to cause diabetes follows.

Influence of Heredity.   That heredity plays a role in caus-ing diabetes has been known for a long time; diabetes seemed to occur in certain families. This holds true even today. Simi-larly, it has been shown that if one identical twin becomes diabetic, there is a great probability that the other will also become diabetic.

Inheritance is a passage of "blueprints" or genes from one generation to another. A gene is an element in the cell that transmits hereditary characteristics and forms a specific part of a response that is carried on from cell to cell. This occurs through a chemical called DNA, which is contained in the chromosomes that are found in the nucleus of the cell. Thus, when the mother's 23 chromosomes and the father's 23 chromosomes combine, they form 46 chromosomes, plus the expression of the sex as determined by the "x" and "y" chromosomes. These chromosomes have the ability to give highly specific information to all body cells. As the fertilized egg cell begins to divide and multiply, the original 48 total chromosomes result in an organism with a specific sex, organ structure, eye and hair color, and the other individual characteristics of life.

For example, if both parents have blue eyes, all their children would theoretically have blue eyes. This would be a condition in which the genes of both parents are expressed in the children. However, if one parent has brown eyes and the other has blue eyes, and if all the children from this mating have brown eyes, one would say that the gene for brown eyes was *dominant*. On the other hand, if both parents had brown eyes and some of the children had blue eyes, one would say that the gene for the blue eyes was *recessive*. Thus, in the mixture of genes from both parents, the gene for brown eyes was usually stronger than that for blue eyes, but the gene for blue eyes could find expression in some genetic combination, resulting in some children with blue eyes.

For years, the genetics of diabetes has been widely discussed and all types of inheritance have been considered. No single gene theory has been compatible with the data known to date. For example, if both parents are diabetic, it is estimated that the children have only a 30% chance of eventually becoming diabetic. Twin studies indicate that a definite genetic component exists in diabetes, but even this is not an absolute rule. Current thinking concerning the inheritance of diabetes postulates that many causes may be responsible for the condition. The exact genetic make-up is unknown, but it is nevertheless important. Interestingly, 12% of newly diagnosed diabetics have close relatives with diabetes, while in the general population, only 2% of normal individuals have relatives with diabetes. One factor operating here is that we do not always know what diseases our ancestors had or even what disorders all our current relatives have. In the Oxford, Massachusetts, study, only about 25% of the diagnosed diabetics knew of relatives with diabetes at the start of the study, but after 15 years, nearly 80% of them knew of some relative who had diabetes, either previously undiagnosed, simply unknown or subsequently developed after the initial interview.

The maturity-onset form of diabetes appears to be linked to a set of genes that is responsible for the familial inheritance of the condition, although the environment, also known as "stress," plays an important role. Obesity is probably the most influential factor.

Juvenile-onset diabetes may be related to specific genetic factors, including an immunologic condition involving antigens. An "antigen" is defined as a substance, usually protein in nature, which, when coming in contact with certain tissues, is recognized as foreign and causes a response, usually an immune response. Unless we are an identical twin, we are all different from one another, owing to the differences in our proteins created by our genetic make-ups. These differences in proteins are called antigens, because they provoke the body to react by forming defensive "antibodies." This immune reaction is performed by certain blood cells in our bodies and is important in protecting us when a foreign antigen like a bacteria or a toxin comes into our bloodstream. The body "recognizes" this as a foreign material and forms antibodies to destroy it. Insulin itself can be antigenic because it may stimulate the formation and release of antibodies which may in turn help make the insulin much less effective.

Recently, attempts at organ transplants have led to the development of a new scientific approach to identify antigens. This is called "typing." With typing, scientists attempt to find people with as many similar (histocompatible) sites or body cells as possible; the process is similar to finding people with like blood types, such as A, B, O, AB, and Rh positive and negative. Cells have many different antigen types, and two specific types, HLA-B8 and HLA-BW15, were recently discovered to be more common in juvenile-onset diabetics than in the general population. However, maturity-onset diabetics seem to have no differences from the general population. From this information, the concept originated that juvenile-onset and maturity-onset diabetes are different diseases, although both appear in the same families much more often than in the general population. The HLA antigen sites may serve as markers, which may be helpful to us in future studies to identify individuals most likely to become diabetic. Putting a flag on your car radio antenna in order to find your car in a full parking lot provides a good analogy for the use of markers in scientific research.

Influence of Viruses. The possibility that viruses may be linked to the onset of diabetes has been considered for a long time. In 1864, a Norwegian scientist reported that a patient developed diabetes following a mumps infection. Another study implicating a mumps virus as a cause of diabetes was reported in Sweden, where the incidence of diabetes following a mumps epidemic was greater than expected. However, other attempts to find a relationship in a variety of studies had not been as fruitful, until English scientists noted a relationship between a strain of viruses known as Coxsackie and diabetes in children. Cases of diabetes in England were more frequent during the winter months as compared to summer, with a similar finding for cases of virus infections. When the British Diabetic Association reported the incidence of new cases of juvenile diabetes, they noticed a great incidence at about four to five years of age and an even higher incidence at 12 to 13 years of age. They postulated that at these ages the children were exposed to various new viruses in primary and secondary schools. Some researchers have found that when certain viruses (encephalomyocarditis virus, EMC) are given to specific strains of mice, the animals become diabetic.

Since the virus would probably affect only certain but not all beta cells, the beta cell infection might possibly cause an antigen-antibody reaction in the circulation. Other diseases of self-destruction of the body have been known for some time. For instance, thyroiditis is a disease in which an infection of the thyroid gland causes the body to produce antibodies (again, protein produced by the body in an attempt to rid it of foreign tissue or antigen) against its own thyroid gland. Recently, antibodies against the beta cell have been found in some diabetics. Thus, we may have the same type of problem in diabetes—the beta cells become a self-destructing mechanism.

To summarize the roles of heredity, immune reactions and infection in causing diabetes, suppose that an individual who is considered susceptible to diabetes, because he has the antigens HLA-B8 and HLA-BW15, becomes infected by a virus that causes beta cell destruction. The dead beta cells act as antigens. Antibodies are produced, because the former beta cells are now considered to be foreign, an enemy. The antibodies go to the remaining beta cells and destroy all of them. Such a theory has some scientific support, and it may prove to be a possible sequence of events causing diabetes in some circumstances. Whereas this theory may afford the possibility of prevention through vaccination, at least 20 different virus-like bodies have been identified that are capable of producing this effect. This makes possible vaccine development difficult.

The Role of Obesity. Although heredity may help to predict the possibility of diabetes, we also know that heredity is important in obesity. Studies have shown that the incidence of obesity when both parents are overweight is 70 to 80%. However, the incidence of obesity is much smaller when both parents are thin, so there may be a genetic predisposition to overweight as well. Similarly, we know that one of the complications of obesity is diabetes. If we were to select randomly 100 new diabetics, 80% would be obese. Many obese diabetics have normal blood sugar levels when they lose weight. Obesity and diabetes also appear to be related in that overweight is associated with a decrease in the activity of insulin in various tissues (e.g., fat and muscle cells). Whereas the beta cells may be secreting large amounts of insulin in an attempt to take care of the food ingested and to maintain the storage of fuels, eventually an insulin shortage occurs because the beta cells are unable to keep up with the demand for insulin necessary to do the job. This situation is often corrected if weight is lost.

Effect of Aging. The incidence of diabetes also appears to be related to increasing age, except the juvenile-onset group. Although the English studies seem to show that juvenile-onset diabetes has its highest incidence starting at age 4 or 5 and reaching a peak in early adolescence, the older-onset diabetes has a high incidence after age 40 and glucose tolerance decreases somewhat with the increasing age of the individual, who may become more "diabetic." This increasing incidence with age may be related to a general decrease in body functions that occurs in all cells with aging.

Effect of Diet. An interesting correlation exists between the types of food eaten and the onset of diabetes. For instance, Yemenite Jews, who had a low incidence of diabetes while eating a very high protein and low carbohydrate diet, appear to have a much higher incidence of diabetes when exposed to a Western civilization diet consisting of more refined sugars and a higher carbohydrate content. Also, in wealthier communities, the incidence of diabetes seems to increase with the degree of wealth. In African communities, diabetes among the natives is rare until high starch and refined foods are eaten. The use of fiber in the diet has been suggested as a possible factor, since high fiber content decreases the incidence of diabetes. The exact mechanism of the role of diet in the onset of diabetes is unknown, but the evidence implicating diet is highly suggestive.

Influence of Hormones. Many hormones circulate in animals, including humans. Examples include sex hormones, hormones produced by the pituitary (a gland located in the middle of the skull below the brain), hormones from the adrenals (glands that sit on top of the kidneys) and others. Although these hormones appear in the circulation in closely regulated amounts, occasionally overproduction by the glands causes higher levels to occur. Excess amounts of growth hormone (from the pituitary) will counteract the activity of insulin and may produce a diabetes-like condition in addition to excess growth. The situation is like someone trying to get into a doorway while others are trying to leave by the same opening. Hormonal imbalance may affect the action of insulin, because thyroid hormone, epinephrine, cortisone and glucagon as well as growth hormone tend to make it less effective. Recently, another hormone, found mostly in the base of the brain, has been described. This substance, somatostatin, presently used as a research tool, appears to block the release of glucagon and anterior pituitary hormone and thus aid insulin function. It has a short effective life, and in research studies it is given only by vein. When somatostatin is effective, the insulin requirement may be greatly reduced.

Influence of Drugs and Medications. Other compounds influence the pancreas. For instance, diuretics are used to decrease blood pressure by decreasing the amount of sodium in the blood, which causes the loss of excess fluids. Simultaneously, another chemical, potassium, may be lost. While the loss of sodium may be beneficial, the loss of potassium is not. These diuretic agents may inadvertently increase the blood sugar level so that diabetes appears to be present. Sometimes simply treating with potassium will return the blood sugar to normal levels. The oral contraceptive agents (birth control pills) seem to raise blood sugar levels by somehow interfering with insulin availability. These compounds usually do not cause diabetes in the nondiabetes-prone person, but they sometimes appear to increase the tendency to diabetes or at least to aggravate it.

Thyroid hormone increases cellular metabolism, thereby increasing the amount of insulin required. Cortisone, a product of the adrenal gland, increases the level of blood glucose and has an antipancreatic influence. These and other substances, such as medications that have an anti-insulin effect, are listed on page 101.

Influence of Illness. In certain diseases, such as inflammation of the pancreas (pancreatitis), following a heart attack or even in the presence of any infection, an elevated blood glucose level may be found. These patients, who have no previous history of diabetes, often return to normal blood glucose levels once the infection or stress has been removed. On the other hand, sometimes diabetes really develops or a diabetic state is unmasked which, if persisting, requires treatment.

Sometimes during such stress, more glucagon may be released, making insulin less effective. It was once believed that elevated blood sugar levels provided a better breeding place for germs. This is probably not true, except perhaps when much sugar is present in the urine. However, observers have noted that phagocytes, a type of white blood cell that serves as a defense for the body by engulfing bacteria, work poorly in the presence of elevated blood sugar levels. Indeed, if the elevated level of blood glucose was maintained, the phagocytes not only slowed down but stopped their usual combat against hostile germs. This permits infection to get the upper hand and promotes even greater stress.

The Effect of Stress.   Many talk about "stress diabetes" as if it were some special form of the disease. Just what role does stress play in the onset of diabetes? The addition of *stress* to *heredity* in the onset of diabetes has been expressed in the statement that "heredity loads the gun while stress pulls the trigger." Many types of stress appear to hurry the onset of diabetes in persons predisposed to it. Aging with its decrease in insulin output may be a factor. In addition to infection and others previously mentioned, another stress factor might be multiple childbirth. The incidence of diabetes increases in women with increased numbers of offspring. For example, a study in South Africa noted that women with more than six children, had a higher incidence of diabetes than those with smaller families. It has been known for some time that women who give birth to exceptionally large babies are more prone to develop future diabetes than those with normal-sized or smaller babies. Unquestionably, stress can play a role, but according to present thinking, stress of itself does not bring on diabetes unless the person is diabetes-prone by heredity (or by earlier viral infections?).

This brings up a point often made by patients who blame the onset of their diabetes on a specific, acute stress, such as an auto accident, an injury, or emotional stress. Unless a blow to the abdomen is so severe as to utterly destroy the pancreas—a difficult situation to survive—the likelihood is that circumstances surrounding the accident and the testing in the hospital probably unmasked an incipient diabetes that was already present. Mental stress has never been shown to cause diabetes. In acute stress situations, such as the recognition of instant danger, some adrenalin is released. This does raise the blood sugar level by preparing the individual for "fight or flight," but this effect is short in duration and constitutes preparation for the emergency. In stress of longer duration, cortisone may be released, which has an anti-insulin effect. However, these situations are self-limited, and if the stress continues, the body response lessens as the person becomes used to the "stress" situation.

Other Factors.   Although a variety of other factors may play a role in the onset of diabetes, suffice to say that we are still probably only touching the top of the iceberg with regard to our knowledge of the exact causes and the role of other factors that influence the onset of diabetes. Toxins in the diet, the body's metabolism or an autonomous mechanism could all play a greater role than we know.

how do I know whether I have diabetes

Diabetes often has been called "the great imitator," because it may affect every organ in the body and can produce a multitude of varying problems. Diabetes may develop gradually, and the victim may not realize he is drinking a little more water, urinating more frequently, becoming tired or losing weight. These symptoms of diabetes may be unnoticed for a long time. At other times, the symptoms are dramatic and occur rapidly. Tests for diabetes should be performed as early as possible, because early appropriate treatment may curtail complications of the disease. The early symptoms of diabetes can occur in nearly any part of the body, for example, as blurred vision (this is discussed on page 153).

THE SKIN. A common complaint of diabetics is severe itching of the skin, usually in the genital (especially vaginal) or anal area. This can cause severe discomfort. Carbuncles, furuncles and difficulty in healing wounds also may be found. Sometimes the patient with untreated diabetes has very high levels of lipids (fats) in the blood, which may cause small, raised, reddish-yellow lesions on the skin called xanthomas. Some persons with diabetes of long duration have a loss of skin elements, especially in the shin area. This is given the formidable name of necrobiosis lipoidica diabeticorum; it means a destruction of tissue. This symptom usually occurs late. Another finding in diabetes, usually of long duration, is brown spots, like freckles, that appear on the lower extremities. These "shin spots" have little significance except cosmetically.

GYNECOLOGIC PROBLEMS. Not uncommonly, gynecologists find evidence suggesting diabetes. Suspicion may be aroused by the presence of a severe infection with a fungus known as Candida. This infection causes irritation, severe itching of the vagina and sometimes a chronic discharge.

THE NERVOUS SYSTEM.   Although the nerves may be affected early (neuropathy), this most often occurs later in the course of the disease. Symptoms may include numbness, tingling, burning or intense sensitivity in certain areas of the skin. The symptoms may be worse at night. Occasionally a diabetic may complain of blurry vision that disappears when one eye is closed. This is due to a temporary paralysis of one of the nerves of the eye muscles, so that they do not focus equally; it disappears spontaneously in three to six weeks.

General fatigue is probably the commonest early manifestation of diabetes. Being tired, fatigued, weak, "unable to get going," headachy or "nervous" are common. Patients sometimes are misdiagnosed as having depression or some severe emotional upset while actually having symptoms of diabetes. Usually, when the diabetes is diagnosed and treated, these symptoms subside.

These are a few of the possible symptoms of diabetes which people can be aware of prior to its diagnosis. As in the Sherlock Holmes stories, patients as well as their physicians should be looking for some of the clues or symptoms that might suggest the diagnosis of diabetes mellitus.

detection: finding new cases

New diabetics are discovered in many ways. Sometimes the symptoms are so obvious that it is almost impossible to avoid the diagnosis of diabetes. On the other hand, the onset can be so insidious that the diagnosis is unsuspected until either an elevated blood glucose level or sugar in the urine is discovered during the course of a routine examination. During the past several decades, many diabetes suspects have been found during detection drives, usually resulting from the activities of a local diabetes association or medical society. Urine testing is sometimes used to seek out diabetes suspects, but this is not the most sensitive method. Usually, glucose does not appear in the urine until the blood glucose level is approximately 160 to 180 mg. per cent or higher. Such levels are already above normal. With an elevated kidney threshold, the blood glucose level might be even higher without glycosuria. The suspect levels are discussed later in this chapter, but suffice to say that an elevated blood glucose level after a meal or after taking glucose by mouth is probably the earliest common sign of diabetes. This may occur long before symptoms are found.

In 1946, a detection study was done in Oxford, Massachusetts, at which time 3,516 of the 4,983 population were tested for diabetes, using blood and urine glucose examinations. Seventy persons with diabetes were found, as well as many persons whose increased blood glucose levels were not elevated sufficiently to warrant a diagnosis of diabetes. These persons were observed for a period of 12 years after the original study. Those with elevated blood glucose levels after meals or after drinking a glucose solution developed clinical diabetes about ten times more frequently than those in the population whose 1946 blood glucose levels had remained within normal limits in spite of the same provocation. An elevated blood glucose level after the stress of glucose suggests that the beta cells have difficulty in releasing enough insulin soon enough, and this may indeed be an indication of early diabetes. A diagnosis, of course, would not be based on a single blood glucose level, even if abnormal. The screening level used in looking for new diabetics is lower than the diagnostic level but it helps to determine those persons most likely to become diabetic. This is a difference between *screening* and *diagnostic* standards for blood glucose levels.

Blood Glucose. At present, the diagnosis of diabetes is made when the blood sugar is elevated above the diagnostic level. Patients often ask, "Do I have any sugar (glucose) in my blood?" The answer is always "Yes," because everyone has blood sugar. The abnormality is a significantly elevated blood glucose level. Ordinarily, the glucose in the blood keeps within a very definite range. When *fasting*, this is between 50 and 100 mg. per cent. After the ingestion of food, or after a challenge to beta cell output by ingestion of glucose, the blood glucose level may become elevated for an hour or so, but will almost never increase above 150 mg. per cent. Normally the blood glucose drops quite rapidly, so that at three hours after the meal, the previous fasting blood glucose levels are reached. *Figure 13* shows the results of a standard 100-gram glucose tolerance test. The standards used are those of whole venous blood—"true glucose" values. Anything consistently above these levels is presumed to represent diabetes mellitus. Al-

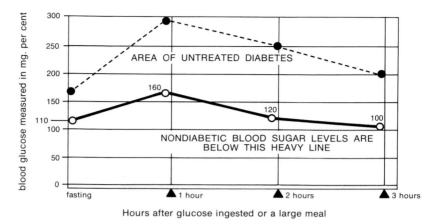

FIG. 13. The glucose tolerance test is usually diagnostic of diabetes; it shows the blood sugar response to an appropriate amount of glucose given by mouth. (These values presume the measurement of "true" glucose methods using whole blood taken from a vein. The values are higher when arterial blood or blood plasma are used for testing.)

though other reasons may exist for elevated blood sugar, these occur less frequently than diabetes and can be ruled out by the physician.

Blood samples taken from the ear lobe or finger pad are called capillary blood. The glucose levels of these samples are usually 20 to 30 mg. per cent higher than that from a vein, if samples are taken an hour or two after eating. This occurs because the capillaries have arterial blood containing a higher blood glucose content. The veins are returning blood with much less glucose content. In the fasting state, both capillary and venous blood have about the same glucose content. Table 1 shows the upper limits of normal with the different types of blood testing. Different interpretations may be applied to the glucose tolerance test, but a completely positive test would be recognized by nearly everyone, since persons with diabetes usually have blood glucose values far above the diagnostic standards. The "slightly elevated" levels are useful for determining those who are potentially diabetic. Early treatment by weight loss or diet often lowers moderately elevated blood glucose levels to normal. While the foregoing criteria are based

TABLE 1. Diagnostic Levels of Blood Glucose Following 100 Grams of Glucose by Mouth* (in mg. per 100 ml)

	Fasting	1 Hour	2 Hours	3 Hours
Venous Blood† (from arm)	110	160	130	110
Capillary Blood‡ (from earlobe or fingertip)	110	190	150	110

*Standards used to evaluate potential diabetics and to diagnose probable diabetics. The diagnosis of diabetes is never made after only one blood or urine sugar test.
†"True sugar" values.
‡Glucose content of capillary (arterial) blood is usually higher than that from vein if taken one or two hours after ingesting food or glucose.

on *whole blood* testing, when *blood plasma* (the liquid portion of the blood with the red cells removed) is used, the results are about 15% higher. These differences are not important to the patient, since the physician ordering the tests knows which is being used. In summary, a significantly elevated blood glucose level is always abnormal, and if it is sufficiently abnormal, it probably indicates diabetes until proven otherwise.

Urine Glucose. Urine testing for glucose is performed more often than blood sugar testing. However, the test for urine glucose is not as sensitive as the blood glucose test for diagnostic purposes. In general, when blood glucose levels are high enough for one to consider the diagnosis of diabetes, glucose is usually present in the urine. However, all sugar in the urine is not diagnostic of diabetes. Sugars other than glucose sometimes appear, and some people have *renal glycosuria,* in which glucose appears in the urine at a lower-than-usual blood glucose level. Others may have elevated levels of blood sugar and presumed diabetes without the appearance of any glucose in the urine. Remember that, while the peak elevation of glucose in the blood occurs one-half to one hour after eating food or glucose, the increase in urine sugar may not occur until one or two hours after the blood glucose peaks.

how to become a diabetic

In considering the data presented thus far, it is obvious that in spite of the many millions of persons who have done so, it is not easy to become a diabetic. First, it is important to have the proper ancestors, a factor over which we have no choice. Although it has not been proven that grandparents or other relatives with diabetes will ensure anyone's becoming a diabetic, if a strong hereditary influence exists, contracting diabetes does become more probable. Recent information suggesting possible viral origin also confounds the matter. There is some evidence that the hereditary candidate for diabetes may sustain damage to the beta cells after a viral infection, especially during youth. In addition, various stress factors may wield their influence. As people age, some degree of defect often occurs in the insulin-producing mechanism, as shown by occasional elevated blood sugar levels in older persons. (These people do not necessarily become diabetic.) Obesity is another means of diminishing the beta cell output. If a woman has multiple childbirths, or if severe and chronic infections occur in either sex, the odds for possible diabetes increase. If heredity were the sole influence, then it would be anticipated that with both parents diabetic, *all* the offspring would become diabetic. Yet, as shown in Figure 14, this does not always occur. Thus, a combination of heredity plus certain stresses does occur in adult-onset diabetes.

Although ethnic origin, religion or country of birth do not have much direct influence on the onset of diabetes, certain groups do have a higher incidence. Certainly populations who have intermarried for long periods or whose native culture emphasizes rich foods and overweight have an increased potential for diabetes. Being rich or poor does not matter too much, except that the affluent have access to more and richer foods and often develop diabetes more frequently. During World War II, the populations deprived of excess nourishment showed a marked drop in the frequency of both overt diabetes and complications such as diabetic coma. Some countries that have improved their economies during the past several decades are paying a price in increased incidence of diabetes. Now the aging of the world live longer, tend to retire earlier and become less active. As they climb the economic ladder, the underdeveloped countries of the world try to emulate the more

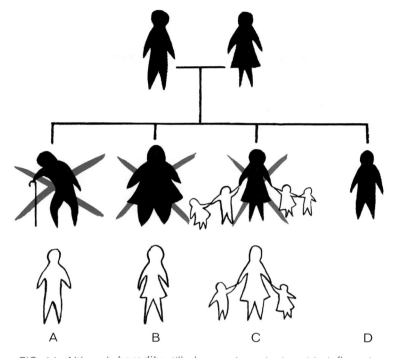

FIG. 14. Although *heredity* still plays an important part in influencing the onset of diabetes, recent studies are less definite about its degree of influence. In the adult-onset diabetic, *stresses* superimposed on the effect of heredity are thought to increase the chances for diabetes to develop. For example, in the past it was thought that if both the mother and the father had diabetes, all their offspring would eventually become diabetic. However, this does not occur. Some reasons why heredity is important but not supreme are illustrated here. *A* might have become a diabetic had he lived to the age of 78, but he only lived until age 70. *B* might have become diabetic if she had weighed 200 lbs., but she never exceeded 140 lbs. *C* might have become diabetic if she had had four children, but she only had two. *D* became diabetic—so that only one of four children developed diabetes.

successful nations. It is not surprising that the diabetes population of the world, as indicated by nearly all surveys, simply grows and grows and grows.

While none of these suggestions can guarantee the onset of diabetes, the data presented indicate that there are definite ways for increasing the opportunities to do so. Avoid those that you can!

Treatment:
General Considerations

The treatment of diabetes, since the first use of insulin in 1922, has been one of the most exciting chapters in the history of medicine. Within our lifetime, the outlook for the diabetic has changed from one of semi-starvation and mere survival to the present status, in which increasing numbers of diabetics have not only lived more than 50 years with their condition, but have lived usefully and well. Although people today are inclined to take much for granted, no one who has lived through the years before and since the discovery of insulin will stop wondering at this miracle that brought the "dead" to life.

The treatment of diabetes usually lasts a lifetime. People not usually disturbed by acute illnesses are often unprepared to cope with the long-term problems posed by diabetes. Treating diabetes is like waging a prolonged war: it is possible to lose some of the battles, but the war must be won. Diabetes is ever-present, and the patient must be treated not only for now but for the future. Travelers on ocean-going vessels have looked at the sea and realized that it is eternally trying to enter the ship. The job of the crew is to keep the sea out, and they are forever scraping, painting, and repairing, because one break in the integrity of the ship's hull could be dangerous. Diabetes is much the same. With modern treatment diabetes can be well-regulated, and this state can be maintained for many more years than was previously thought.

goals of treatment

The goal of diabetes treatment is to restore the patient and his physiology to a state as normal as possible, so that he can live a life as normal as possible. These "as possible's" are compromises made necessary by the presently available methods of treatment, which are not yet perfect. Some claim to be unconcerned about blood glucose levels or the amount of sugar wasted in the urine. Yet many people simply do not feel well when their diabetes is inadequately treated. Few persons really can feel well if they are losing much of their food intake, which should provide nourishment, by squandering large amounts of glucose in the urine. Some patients, after getting their diabetes well-regulated, express amazement because they had felt miserable for so long that they considered the misery normal. They had forgotten how well they could feel.

In some patients, maintaining a normal level of blood sugar at all times is difficult. This does not mean that the goal is not important, but that it may take a greater effort. The *ideal* (as in the nondiabetic person) is for the diabetic always to have normal blood glucose levels and urine free of sugar. Along with this, there should be no elevated levels of blood fats or other abnormal blood chemistry. This is the ideal; if one aims lower, the end result is almost certain to be worse.

the "normal" life

It has sometimes been said that the diabetic can live a "normal" life. This is not strictly true. Any person who has to think always of *what* and *when* and *how much* he eats, who must do urine sugar tests regularly and who must use insulin injections once or twice daily cannot be said to live a "normal" life. For most people, a "normal" life means doing what they please without thought of medicines, diet or other restraints. The diabetic life, while not "normal," can be extremely livable, useful and enjoyable. Over the past 50 years many thousands of diabetics worldwide have achieved great things in every walk of life. Many of them are free of significant complications after many years of insulin-requiring diabetes.

> DIET—INSULIN—ORAL HYPOGLYCEMIC AGENTS —EXERCISE are the only available means for treating diabetes today. How these will be used in treatment is an individual matter, depending on the patient and as determined by the physician.

essentials of treatment

The chief items in the treatment of diabetes are diet, insulin, oral agents and exercise. Each of these depends basically on the use of insulin, produced either by the patient's own pancreas or given by injection.

THE PLACE OF DIET. Control of the type and amount of food ingested continues as the basis of all treatment of diabetes. A large percentage of patients who develop diabetes in middle and later life retain the ability to make insulin to some extent. This insulin, although not enough to permit a completely free diet, may be adequate if the amount and type of food are adjusted and brought into relationship with physical activity. Consequently, if a diet or eating plan, adjusted to the person's need, is followed and excess body weight reduced, satisfactory regulation of diabetes may be attained.

USE OF INSULIN. If the available body insulin is not adequate, and if more is needed in spite of careful diet, it may be necessary to use insulin given by injection.

ORAL AGENTS. During the last 20 years, certain tablets have been used by many diabetics, and these agents enable the patient's own pancreas to increase the available insulin at least for a time. They are effective only if the pancreas is capable of responding to stimulation. When this mechanism is effective, patients use their own body insulin to meet their needs. In addition to the compounds that stimulate the release of insulin, other mechanisms are effective.

EXERCISE. This is important to the diabetic because, in addition to improving muscle tone and strength, it may reduce the insulin requirement.

These are the main tools of treatment now. Which will the physician prescribe? In many persons with adult-onset diabetes who are overweight, diet alone may be most effective. If not, sometimes the addition of an oral agent may help. On the other hand, young diabetics nearly always require insulin as indeed, do many adult-onset diabetics. Often treatment with oral agents becomes less effective after a period and may need to be replaced by insulin.

Whatever the means of treatment, it always involves insulin, whether it comes from the patient's own "homemade" supply, is stimulated or aided by oral compounds or is injected insulin from animal sources. Many new patients ask "Will I have to take insulin for the rest of my life?" This is not easy to predict. Most patients who initially need insulin may require injections for the rest of their lives, not because it is habit-forming, but because they are unable to make enough of their own and therefore will always need to replace it. With optimal treatment, older patients sometimes are able to reduce their insulin dose or even return to diet treatment alone.

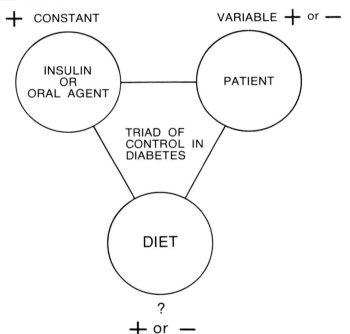

FIG. 15. Triad of control in diabetes. The *dose* of insulin or oral hypoglycemic agent is usually *constant*. Generally, if a patient injects 20 units of insulin, he gets 20 units of effect.

The *patient* is usually an *inconstant* factor. His activity, emotional state, and even vital signs change, depending on many factors.

The importance of *diet* in control becomes obvious. If the diet is *inconstant*, then two factors out of three are variable and regulation of the diabetes may be difficult. On the other hand, if the diet is a *constant and dependable* factor, the chances for good control obviously improve.

balanced treatment

The treatment of diabetes must be in balance. Too much food may increase the insulin requirement. Less food or more exercise may reduce the blood glucose level. Actually, as shown in Figure 15, the control of diabetes has three componants: (1) the patient, who at best is often inconstant; (2) the daily injection of insulin or the administration of oral agents, which is a fairly constant influence; (3) diet. If diet is observed well, then two of the three influences on control are constant and there is a reasonably good chance for regulation of the diabetes. On the other hand, if diet is ignored, then the chances for regulation are dim indeed.

3

Diet

As pointed out earlier, food is fuel for the body, just as gasoline or another combustible liquid is fuel for the machine. Both man and machine depend on fuel in order to function. In man, the need for adequate food is especially important because, in addition to its use as fuel, it also supplies the ingredients to replace body parts as they wear out. Moreover, man has the ability to store fuel not immediately used in depots in his body for future use. The need for fuel varies according to body activity, climate and basal energy requirements of each individual. These needs may change from day to day and sometimes from minute to minute. The energy requirements of the average normal adult during a 24-hour period are about 25 calories per kilogram or 11 calories per pound of ideal body weight. Each bit of energy used demands more calories and marked physical activity raises the requirement.

All food consists of carbohydrate, protein and fat. Food also contains vitamins and minerals. Rarely do people eating a well-balanced diet require extra amounts of these.

1. *Carbohydrate* is needed for energy and produces four calories for each gram eaten.
2. *Protein* is needed for a slower, more sustained form of energy release and to build muscle and tissue. Each gram also produces four calories.
3. *Fat* provides energy and when stored, a depot for future energy needs. Each gram of fat yields nine calories.

The diet, for both diabetic and nondiabetic, should be chosen according to individual needs. A thin, active person in a cold climate may need many more calories than a heavy, inactive individual. Adults in sedentary occupations may only require between 1000 and 1500 calories daily, while active or growing persons may require 2500 to 3000 or more calories daily. People trying to lose weight may have to cut their intake to below 1000 calories per day. Growing children require much higher levels of calories than most relatively inactive adults, particularly those calories supplied by protein.

is diet obsolete

"Diet" is one of the most unpopular words in any language. Mere mention of the word suggests sacrificing the good things in life that people most enjoy. The idea of dieting attacks mankind's basic instincts. The young enjoy goodies and even childhood poetry notes that "visions of sugar plums danced in their heads." Dieting is no pleasanter for older persons, among whom are many of the world's diabetics. When their age deprives them of many other pleasures, they naturally resist the loss of one of their great remaining joys, eating things they like.

With the availability of insulin and the oral hypoglycemic agents, many wonder, "Is diet now obsolete?" Why even consider changing eating patterns? The fact is that diet is more important now than ever before. Most modern means of treatment require that the physician estimate 24 hours in advance what the insulin or oral agent dose should be. The diet must take into consideration both the dosage of insulin or oral agent and the patient's physical activities. Success or failure with any agent that lowers blood sugar levels hinges on dietary adherence. Thus, diet is not obsolete. It is, in fact, now receiving greater attention than ever before, and justifiably so.

what is diet

For the diabetic, a diet is simply a combination and balancing of those nutritious foods that will enable him to keep and use these foods for his energy needs. The goal is not food deprivation, but rather an adjustment of eating habits to fit individual needs. Every diabetic diet should be tailor-made and must consider the patient's height, weight, type of activities, medication and also personal likes and dislikes. The diet should be outlined as simply as possible, commensurate with the patient's understanding, ability and desires.

Many people without diabetes observe a diet of one kind or another, whether to lose weight, to gain weight, to restrict salt, or to treat duodenal ulcer, gout and many other medical conditions. The diabetic is no longer unique because of the necessity to diet.

The basic purpose of the diet prescription is to provide an adequate, usable and nourishing food intake. The person with maturity-onset diabetes has a short supply of insulin. An appropriate diet that does not overtax his limited insulin-producing capacity may enable him to do very well. Except in juvenile-onset cases or in emergencies that obviously require insulin injections, an adequate trial with diet alone is the first treatment of choice. However, it may soon be apparent that injected insulin or an oral blood-sugar-lowering agent is needed to assist the patient's own insulin production. The dosage of insulin or other medication must be chosen deliberately. Its utilization is influenced by food, exercise, the effect of other endocrine hormones and many other factors. Bearing all this in mind, the following diet principles are enumerated.

1. *The food intake must be spread throughout the waking part of the day.* If all the food were eaten at one time, the insulin would be inadequate, resulting in elevated blood glucose levels and glucose in the urine. During the rest of the day, the patient might develop low blood sugar reactions. For this reason, the diet is often divided into portions, with one-fifth of the calories to be taken at breakfast, two-fifths at lunch and two-fifths at the evening meal, usually with small snacks in between. This program is adjusted according to the work and activity habits of the patient.

2. *The diet must provide balanced proportions of carbohydrate, protein and fat.* Some foods (such as carbohydrates) break down into energy very rapidly; proteins and fats are used more slowly. Of the carbohydrates, some are utilized more quickly than others. Most sweets are broken down and absorbed too quickly to be used in the body of the diabetic and are lost in the urine.

3. *The diet must provide all of the elements needed for good nutrition.*

4. *The diet should provide approximately the same amount of food each day in order to maintain stability.* Extra nourishment is allowed for those periods when extra energy is needed.

tools of diet

The tools used to construct a diet are simple. No matter what anyone eats, the only available foods are composed of carbohydrate, protein and fat. The *carbohydrates* provide a fast fuel for body energy. Highest in carbohydrate are sugar, candy, syrup, sweets and pastries. High-starch foods include bread, crackers, potatoes, rice, cereals, beans, corn, macaroni, milk, and similar products. Fruit and vegetables also contain varying amounts of carbohydrate. Carbohydrate foods are the least expensive and most easily available foods throughout the world. The *proteins* include meat, fish, fowl, cheese and eggs. They provide a slower form of energy and also provide the building blocks for body replacement. Although carbohydrate eventually breaks down to glucose, proteins become amino acids. The *fats* provide an even slower form of energy and break down to fatty acids. These are stored when they are not quickly utilized for energy. Fatty foods include butter, margarine, cream, fat of meat, bacon, oils, mayonnaise, and all fried foods. Although fat-rich foods are often most delicious, gram for gram they are more than twice as high in calories as carbohydrates and proteins.

The body also needs vitamins and minerals, which are discussed later.

planning the diet

When the carbohydrate, protein and fat are used or metabolized by the body, they produce energy measured as calories. In spite of articles to the contrary, unfortunately calories *do count* and probably constitute the first consideration in planning any diet, including a diabetic diet. Whether you yawn or run up a hill, you use some energy or calories.

There are many ways of determining the calories needed. One method of estimating the daily requirement is to determine what the ideal weight should be and adjusting the calories accordingly. Choosing the daily food intake according to physical activity is also useful. Table 12 (p. 124) has a list of activities and the approximate number of calories used during each. A good diet provides the ideal number of calories for the

individual's needs. Few persons have exactly the same requirements.

Diet Building. Certain rules of nutrition must be followed
in planning a diet for a diabetic. For example, one gram of
protein is needed for each kilogram (2.2 pounds) of ideal body
weight. For growing children, much larger amounts—2 to 4
grams per kilogram—are necessary. In general, the diet should
contain between 60 and 100 grams of protein daily. *Carbohydrate* needs vary according to the individual, but in general,
satisfactory amounts for the diabetic range from 150 to 250
grams or more a day. *Fat* must be estimated carefully because
it provides the most calories per gram, and if not used, it
remains in storage. Increasingly, studies show a need for less
fat. The fat in the diet is determined by the desired weight of
the diabetic. Growing children, of course, can use relatively
larger amounts of fat. It is possible to prescribe a balanced diet
providing fewer than 1000 calories a day for the person who
must lose weight and one providing many more calories for an
especially active person.

The diabetic diet is simply a modified eating plan using
ordinary foods. All members of the family can eat the diet
because no "special" foods are used. Large amounts of carbohydrates, especially sweets and pastries, are avoided, but the
patient's likes, dislikes and food habits are considered. If some
prefer pasta or others rice, these may be used as bread and
potato substitutes, but the quantity used must be carefully
watched. Further instructions for calculating diet are given in
Appendix 2.

The amount of carbohydrate prescribed today is more
liberal than previously. Candy, sweets, pastries and other
foods high in sugar must be avoided completely because they
are absorbed so quickly into the bloodstream with such a
precipitous rise in blood glucose that the available insulin
cannot cope with them, and they are promptly wasted in the
urine. However, as discussed later, sugar-containing foods
may be used to prevent or treat low blood sugar reactions
resulting from too much insulin or unusually vigorous exercise. Thus, not only is the kind of food important, but also how
much is retained in the body. It is amazing how much more
food people eat than they realize. One reason for the perpetual

TABLE 2. Standards of Diet Adherence

Classification	Characteristics
Free Diet	No restrictions; patient eats everything, including sweets and pastries.
Poor	Avoidance of sweets and pastries, but otherwise diet is variable and in general unrestricted.
Fair	Estimation of quantities of food with avoidance of sweets and pastries and excesses of carbohydrate-rich food, but frequent dietary indiscretions.
Good	Generally careful adherence to diet with weighing and/or measuring food not less than once a month, but with occasional dietary indiscretions.
Excellent	Careful adherence with weighing and/or measuring food not less than once a week and almost never a dietary indiscretion.

hunger and fatigue of people with unregulated or uncontrolled diabetes is that often vast amounts of glucose are lost in the urine. How closely a person follows his diet, or how closely he should follow it, varies with the individual and the objectives of his physician. Table 2 shows a general classification of diet adherence used at the Joslin Clinic.

In diet building:

1. A choice is made regarding the total amount of calories required. Through trial and error, the diet is gradually adjusted to the individual's needs. This requires close cooperation between doctor and patient.

2. Personal preferences and habits must be taken into account. Of the total number of calories chosen, 40% may come from carbohydrate, 20% from protein and 40% from fat. The proportions may vary according to the individual physician's inclinations as well as the patient's condition and cooperation. In recent years, the tendency has been to prescribe diets that are more generous in carbohydrate (45 to 50% of calories) and lower in fat. As far as practicable, polyunsaturated fats of vegetable origin should be used in preference to animal fats (see p. 64). In general, certain foods that are difficult for the diabetic to utilize are best avoided entirely (Table 3).

TABLE 3. Foods Likely to Cause Problems

In general, these foods should not be used in a diabetic diet unless approved by the physician or in case of hypoglycemic (low blood sugar) reaction due to insulin:

Alcohol	Kool-Aid, regular
Bacon and sausage, maple-flavored	Marmalade
Bread, fruit, nut or gluten	Molasses
Cake	Muffins, fruit or nut
Candy	Pastries
Cereals, sugar-coated	Pie
Cookies, frosted	Potatoes (escalloped)
Creamed foods or sauces	Preserves
Dates	Puddings
"Dietetic" foods (see Appendix 5)	Raisins
Doughnuts	Scrapple
Deep-fried foods (unless fat	Sherbet
deducted)	Snow Balls
Gelatin desserts, regular	Soda, tonic, pop, and other usual
Gravies	soft drinks, regular and some diet
Gum, regular or candy-coated	drinks (see Appendix 5)
Honey	Sugar
Ice Cream	Sundaes
Ice Milk	Syrups
Jam	Yogurt (fruited)
Jelly	

Food Substitutions. Life would be dull indeed without changes in clothes and colors and most certainly without variety of foods. Although eating a medium orange as dessert is perfectly acceptable, this might become tiresome if repeated every day. As shown in Appendix 2, hosts of possible substitutes are available. For the medium orange, a small apple, $1\frac{1}{2}$ cups of tomato juice, three peach halves or one-half of a medium-sized honeydew melon may be substituted. Almost anything on the diet can be substituted by another food of the same category. For example, those who struggle with children and their dietary peculiarities should be comforted to know that one tablespoonful of peanut butter is approximately equal in nourishment to one ounce of beef or one medium egg, keeping in mind that the peanut butter is rich in carbohydrate and fat as well. Fortunately, children require more carbohydrate. The enjoyment of any eating plan depends on one's knowledge and cleverness in exchanging one food for another that may be preferred. Thus, varied and nutritious menus are always possible, and indeed superb gourmet recipes are available for diabetics who are inclined to such delights.

Eating on Sick Days.   Unfortunately, even diabetics become ill at times. On such occasions, those who use insulin still require it and indeed may need larger doses (see p. 303). Eating the usual solid foods may be impossible, however, and it is best not to try to force-feed if nausea and vomiting occur. When liquids can be retained, broths, clear soups or tea with sugar (for nourishment) should be sipped slowly every hour, although not necessarily in large amounts. Under these circumstances, regular ginger ale (not the low-calorie type) may be used to provide needed carbohydrate. Patients often mistakenly attempt large feedings that are not retained, in which case even a mouthful of liquid, such as sweetened tea or ginger ale, if kept down and repeated every 20 minutes, is preferable. In severe illness with dehydration, it may be necessary to give fluids intravenously; this would be arranged by your personal physician.

Ethnic Diets.   Diabetes is a worldwide condition and fortunately it is perfectly possible to diet in any culture and be reasonably happy. After all, a meatball pizza is nothing more than carbohydrate, protein and fat with possibly some specially flavored sauce. A bagel provides 120 calories and lox (smoked salmon), 25 calories per half ounce. A matzo ball weighing 15 grams (about $\frac{1}{2}$ ounce) can be had for 55 calories. All the world has contributed to our culture, and many Americans prefer the ethnic foods they have long enjoyed, whether they be borscht, tacos or Einlauf soup. All foods, regardless of method of preparation, are only carbohydrate, protein and fat.

Dining Out.   One of life's great pleasures is that of eating some place other than home. A few restaurants now use menus that state caloric values, but even without these, there is no reason why, with care, a good meal cannot be enjoyed. Although exceptions to the rules may occur during periods of intense physical activity, such as skiing or swimming, good general rules for eating out appear on page 55. A more comprehensive guide is found in Appendix 3.

DINING OUT

Once you are familiar with your diet plan, can accurately estimate sizes of portions, and have a knowledge of substitution, you are ready to dine out. BASIC GUIDELINES FOR SUCCESS:

1. Know the preparation of the dish you are ordering.
2. Know the ingredients of the dish.
3. Ask for salad dressing separate from salad for accurate substituting.
4. Beware of foreign sugar substitutes. Bring a familiar brand with you.
5. Don't assume anything! If you don't know, ask!

The Weighed Diet. Many roads may lead to the same destination, and certainly different approaches lead to diet regulation. Although some of these may differ from the practice of the Joslin Clinic, many are quite satisfactory. A diet must be tailored to the motivation and understanding of the person using it. Obviously, the most accurate method is to weigh, measure or carefully estimate food portions. Weighing food is a good training procedure early in the course of diabetes until the eye and hand have learned to judge amounts of food. Some patients are not inconvenienced by weighing much of the time; others learn to estimate quite accurately. Some weigh portions at intervals as a form of retraining. However, weighing should be regarded as a means to an end rather than an end in itself. Any means of achieving a suitable and nutritious diet is acceptable. Learning a building-block method, using set amounts of carbohydrates, proteins and fats and then adding food blocks to make up the diet prescription is not hard. Substituting is not too difficult.

The ADA Diet. Since 1950, many physicians and dietitians have used a system of teaching diet as outlined in the booklet entitled "Exchange Lists for Meal Planning," prepared by committees of the American Diabetes Association, the American Dietetic Association and the U.S. Public Health Service. Many thousands of these are in use. With this plan, all foods are divided into six groups called exchange lists. Each food in a list contains about the same amounts of carbohydrate, protein and fat as any other food in that group. The patient is instructed regarding the number of exchanges to take from the various lists for the three main meals and in-between snacks. For this system to work, both the patient and his doctor must know exactly what is prescribed. For example, if the patient is to have Meal Plan No. 3, he should know that this is an 1800-calorie diet, and also that it contains approximately 180 grams of carbohydrate, 80 grams of protein and 80 grams of fat, as well as the specific foods employed in each exchange list. This diet uses household measures. As with any other regimen, probably the most important ingredient in its success is the patient's desire. This American Diabetes Association booklet, "Exchange Lists for Meal Planning," has been revised recently and may be obtained from their headquarters (600 Fifth Avenue, New York, N.Y. 10020).

Other Diets.   Basically, only four diet choices are available. (1) There is a completely unrestricted diet, as practiced by many nondiabetics. This can be good or hopelessly poor. An example of an extremely poor diet is the not uncommon practice of teenagers stopping for "breakfast" at a lunch counter and ordering sugar doughnuts and a Coke. However, not too many diabetics or nondiabetics actually follow a completely unrestricted diet. Most people do not continuously eat as much of everything as often as strikes their fancy. Certainly diabetics with any degree of instability cannot survive such a regimen without taking overwhelming amounts of insulin, which must be constantly juggled in a futile attempt to cover the capricious and excessive food intake. (2) There is a so-called "free" diet, in which nothing is measured and the types of food are unrestricted except for the exclusion of large amounts of fast-acting carbohydrate or sugar-containing foods. Some patients with the mildest diabetes survive with such nonplanned meals. Usually they are very active, keep their weight down and have considerable insulin-making capability. (3) An estimated diet can be quite accurate if the patient has had good basic training and is familiar with approximate food equivalents. (4) Weighed or measured diets are the ultimate ideal. Although many patients will not choose this discipline, many successfully do so, perhaps with some modifications.

diet results

The results of diet regulation can be astounding. Many people, whose diabetes was so irregular that they were always on the verge of ketoacidosis or insulin reaction, learned that with a reasonably uniform food intake, their lives ran much more smoothly. Some of the most striking success stories have come from an intelligent, highly motivated group—airplane pilots. Federal regulations prohibit persons from piloting aircraft if they require either insulin or oral hypoglycemic agents. If diabetes is discovered early, often it may be successfully treated with diet. With motivation stemming from an endangered lucrative occupation, diabetic pilots adhere to a diet very carefully and, with frequent supervision, have sometimes extended their careers for a number of years. Incidentally, very few persons with diabetes have successfully survived as long as 40 years without good understanding and reasonable observance of diet.

obesity

Obesity is the plague of today's society. Many excuses are given for obesity, but very few reasons. A common complaint heard by the physician is, "Doc, it must be my glands." This cause of obesity is quite rare. The most common reason for overweight is eating more calories than are used. Whether due to less activity or increased food intake, the tendency to overweight seems to increase with increasing age (Table 4). Sometimes, ethnic factors predominate, because obesity is considered a sign of prosperity and good health in some cultures. Unfortunately, early influences prevail and habits become established. When you see an obese child walking hand-in-hand with an obese mother and obese grandmother, you know that the odds are great that the child will be a loser in the weight race. This results not only from heredity, but from the eating habits of the family group (*Fig. 16*). There are occasional people like the nursery rhyme couple, "Jack Spratt could eat no fat—his wife could eat no lean," but they are the exceptions.

The dangers of overweight are documented elsewhere. The ideal weight is now thought to be slightly less than previous calculations. Ideal weight tables are given in Appendix 4.

TABLE 4. Tendency to Get Fat Increases With Age

	Age	Percentage of persons who exceed ideal weight by 10% or more	Percentage of persons who exceed ideal weight by more than 20%
WOMEN	20–29	23	12
	30–39	41	25
	40–49	59	40
	50–59	67	46
MEN	20–29	31	12
	30–39	53	25
	40–49	60	32
	50–59	63	34

Adapted from Metropolitan Life Insurance Company, studies reported in U.S. News & World Report, 6 June 1965, p. 68.

Losing Weight.   The reason for the "magic" diets now in vogue is that practically none of the special or "fad" diets are successful for any period of time. Fads come and go. Everyone would love to believe that calories don't count. Almost any diet will cause weight loss for a short time. There is no really happy, enjoyable means of losing weight once overweight has been present for any length of time. Many people become overweight early in life. If a person gains as little as two pounds a year, this increase amounts to 40 pounds in 20 years. The former college athlete deludes himself with the thought that he really isn't fat, simply "a bit out of condition." Some of the common plaints are: "I don't know why I am fat; I hardly eat anything" and "I eat like a bird." Some birds, of course, eat two or three times their weight in food each day but get enough violent physical activity in flying that their weight remains normal. Very often hospitalized patients are content with a 1500-calorie diet, when at home much more food did not satisfy them. For one thing, extra food is not easily available in most hospitals and dietitians cleverly provide foods large in bulk but low in value. People who are unhappy, depressed and lonely tend to eat more. Many people nibble snacks and watch television all evening, quitting only to raid the refrigerator once more on the way to bed. Dr. Jean Mayer, noted nutrition authority, states that "all patients are mal-

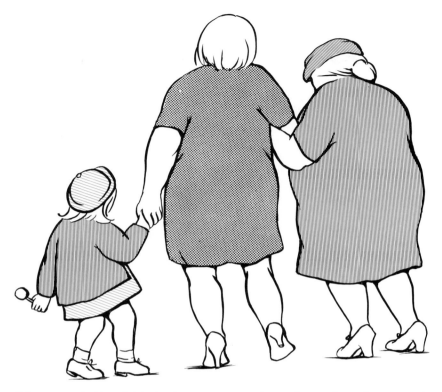

FIG. 16. A chubby child who has an overweight mother and an obese grand-mother will probably become an overweight adult. This cycle can be broken, but ethnic habits and eating patterns often make changing this type of life-style difficult.

nourished until proven otherwise." He means that patients eat not only too much but the wrong foods.

Research has shown that greatly overweight people have an excess number of fat cells, an abnormality that continues in spite of weight loss and is probably caused by overfeeding in early childhood. Drugs, hormones, psychotherapy and even hypnosis have been attempted as aids to weight loss. Studies have shown that because fat cells have decreased sensitivity to insulin, basal insulin levels are not affected by age nearly as much as by overweight. Muscle likewise is less sensitive to insulin when the body is fat. Thus, the need for insulin is clearly increased in the overweight person.

Dr. George Cahill has noted that, just as we ordinarily consume so many meals per day and per year, the average automobile gas tank may be refilled 300 times before the car is junked. However, some people drive around with the tank half empty and others with three or four extra tanks filled to the brim. In similar fashion, the overweight person, in contrast to his slim brother who needs each feeding to keep going, harbors a vast reservoir of energy or calories stored as fat to which he is regularly adding and doesn't use.

If a person is in perfect balance with 2000 calories a day and his activity and exercise keep him at a normal weight, one extra piece of candy (20 calories) is only 1% of the total diet, but this 1% error daily can cause an increase in weight of about two pounds a year.

What is the best way to keep weight down?

1. Lower the calories. A normal 45-year-old man with a sedentary occupation uses about 15 calories per pound of body weight a day. Increasing the expenditure of energy in work or exercise requires a greater caloric intake. Although recent studies show that the average caloric intake per person in the United States is close to 3200 calories a day, this figure would not apply to the middle-aged and elderly segments of the population, from which most diabetics come.

2. Exercise is important. Most people exercise too little.

3. Stay happy and try to avoid depression. Oscar Wilde once said, "When I am in trouble, eating is the only thing that consoles me."

Special Diet Systems—Good and Bad.   About 30% of those who take part in a group weight-reducing program lose 20 pounds or more. Another third lose less than that, while the remaining third fail to lose weight. Unfortunately, after the weight reduction program is completed, much of the weight is frequently gained back, sometimes with interest.

Among the most successful diet programs is Weight Watchers. The founder noted that people had greater success in losing weight when they got together to discuss their mutual problems, much as in other group therapy. The success of Weight Watchers is also based on a high-protein diet. Sessions usually are held weekly. Members are weighed and gains or losses noted. This is not really a crash weight-reduction program; actually, there are nine diets broken down into reducing diets and diets to level off at a desired weight. The goal is to lose approximately 2 to 2½ pounds a week. If diabetics use this program, they must remember that their dosage of insulin or oral agent may need reduction.

Another popular program is TOPS, which means "Take Off Pounds Sensibly." This also is based on group therapy. Diet Workshop was started by overweight housewives who looked at themselves in the mirror, disliked what they saw and did something about it. Basically the program involves a method of changing one's life style and behavior patterns. No foods are completely banned, and indeed the program deliberately allows for "cheating" by underprescribing food so that the alleged "extra" foods with which the dieter may cheat are all part of the program, which is a little less compulsive than some of the others. Again, bear in mind that all these programs were designed for overweight persons in general rather than for diabetics.

In addition to these groups, many "magic" diets abound whose basic soundness is often suspect and which often are unphysiologic. Dr. Yudkin's diet is a very low carbohydrate eating plan in which the patient eliminates most carbohydrate, the largest source of calories. A certain amount of carbohydrate is necessary for diabetics, and if it is reduced too much with an increase in fats and cholesterol, this diet may be harmful in the long run. The cleverly promoted "Drinking Man's Diet" excited popular imagination some years ago and appealed to those who are interested in the "modern" life style. Significant alcohol drinking, particularly for diabetics, creates more problems than it solves, and this diet was condemned by nearly all responsible nutritionists.

Dr. Stillman's high-protein diet consists almost entirely of protein and animal fat. He believes that protein is more difficult to digest and therefore the body uses more energy to do so. The Stillman diet allows the free use of lean meat, poultry, eggs, seafood and certain cheeses. Most dairy and all carbohydrate foods are forbidden. The diet also requires drinking at least two quarts of water a day. A high degree of physical activity is encouraged. Dr. Frederick J. Stare of Harvard refers to this diet as "intentional imbalance of nutrition." Honest scientific questions exist whether a high protein diet, at the cost of everything else, is really healthful and beneficial or even possible on a long-term basis.

Dr. Atkins' program is a recent diet "sensation," praised or condemned by nearly everyone. Many nutritionists have condemned it. The diet starts with no carbohydrate whatsoever but is very high in fat. Gradually, some carbohydrate is added. The weight loss is said to be accomplished by burning fat as measured by the ketones released. In other words, a definite attempt is made to develop ketosis, instead of desperately trying to avoid it as most diabetics do. As a matter of fact, it is a low carbohydrate diet, which releases less insulin. Burning the dieter's own fats as fuel and seeking a state of acidosis as a weight-reducing measure are goals with this diet. Dr. Atkins warns that, in a diabetic, the danger of ketosis becoming acidosis is very real and possibly dangerous.

This type of diet does work for many people. The appetite becomes less after a period; actually, it is a slow starvation. Once again, the problem is the difficulty in long-term use, as well as the fact that many authorities believe that diets high in cholesterol and saturated fats may be harmful. This diet can work for a while, but success with any diet requires a change in lifestyle, and that is not easy to achieve. Along with the "protein-sparing" diet have come promotions of various liquid protein concoctions. The Food and Drug Administration has warned that deaths of unregulated dieters may be related to indiscriminate use of these crash-diet aids.

Many other diets have appeared, taken a brief turn in the spotlight, and then disappeared. Some represent hopeful promises couched in fancy names. Any diet not based on sound nutritional principles or not capable of being followed for long periods of time cannot and should not be attempted by diabetics.

Pills to Lose Weight.   Many people who try to lose weight approach their physician with the plea, "Doc, can I have some pills to lose weight?" Except when a patient has accumulated fluid and needs a diuretic (medication that helps to remove unwanted fluid from the body) or has an inadequately functioning thyroid that requires medication, no pills exist that cause weight to melt away. The only pills that might affect weight are appetite suppressants. Most of these are based on amphetamines (also known as "pep pills" and "uppers") and as such they have been condemned because they may be habit-forming and they overstimulate the nervous system. The Food and Drug Administration and the American Medical

Association Council on Drugs have criticized the use of amphetamines for weight reduction because, in addition to the foregoing, their effect is short-lived. At best, these drugs, if carefully used, provide a temporary crutch for short periods of time only. No magic pill can take the place of a sensible, well-balanced diet.

Artificial Sweeteners.   Although not strictly necessary, artificial sweeteners have made life more bearable for those who crave something sweet but must reduce calories. The best known of these agents have been saccharin and more recently the cyclamates. These chemicals have been widely used for years throughout the world in bakery goods, soft drinks and many other products, and it came as a great shock to diabetics and other diet-conscious persons when, after conflicting opinions and actions, the Food and Drug Administration finally removed cyclamates from the market, first as a food sweetener and then as a diet additive. Huge amounts of cyclamate fed to rats were said to be responsible for causing occasional cases of bladder cancer in some studies. However, the amount of cyclamate fed to the rats was 500 times the maximum recommended for human consumption. Nevertheless, cyclamates were removed from the market because of the Delaney amendment to public law, which states, in simple terms, that anything that might cause cancer in any species of animal, regardless of the relationship, cannot be sold to be used as, or in preparation of, food. The National Academy of Sciences and the National Research Council previously had recommended certain limits on human consumption, stating "Unlimited consumption is not warranted." However, many medical authorities do not agree with the total ban.

Saccharin has been the sweetener most in use since the removal of cyclamate. Recently, the availability of saccharin has been threatened by results of Canadian research, which suggest that long-term studies conducted with massive doses of saccharin fed to laboratory animals indicate an increased risk of bladder cancer. The release of this information by the Food and Drug Administration touched off a public controversy. Because of the Delaney Amendment, the FDA proposed that saccharin be removed from foods but made available over the counter, to diabetics and others who need it for medical purposes, much like vitamins are sold. Most medical circles felt that the attitude of the FDA was clearly an "overkill." The amounts given to the laboratory rats in the study would equal a human consumption of about 600 bottles of saccharin-containing soda pop daily. There is no evidence linking saccharin with cancer in man; moreover, saccharin has been in use since 1879, and no figures suggest any increase in bladder cancer in diabetics. The House Commerce Subcommittee on Health and Environment has voted an 18-month delay until the matter can be settled more definitively. In general, it is felt that the hazards posed to diabetics in eating foods that contain sugar with resulting elevated blood sugar levels are greater than any possible carcinogenic effect of saccharin in the distant future. Meanwhile, other synthetic sweeteners are undergoing trial. One of these, a protein (Aspartame), seems closest to availability. Another preparation (Neo-DHC), made from the bioflavinoids of citrus fruit peelings, has been developed in Israel and is being studied.

fats and cholesterol in the diet

Fats in the diet have been a source of controversy and confusion for many years. Fat is needed as a source of calories and for storage of calories. Excessive fats are harmful because too many calories are provided and stored. Overweight has been linked to many diseases, including heart disease and high blood pressure, as well as atherosclerosis, a condition to which many diabetics are prone.

Dr. Jean Mayer, nutritionist and now president of Tufts University, has been particularly vocal in his criticism of the high fat content in American diets; he is quoted as saying, "It is unfortunate that our federal government, which already dragged its feet to a scandalous extent as regards cigarette smoking, is equally negligent as regards saturated fat."

In 1960, the American Heart Association called for reasonable substitution of polyunsaturated for saturated fats in order to decrease blood cholesterol levels; more recently, it has again strongly recommended decreased intake of saturated fats. However, the Food and Drug Administration has ruled that labeling of food to suggest that dietary substitution of polyunsaturated fats may prevent heart disease is a misdemeanor, and it recently further stated that "manipulation of blood cholesterol levels through diet is not conclusively accepted as the best way to treat or control heart or artery disease." No wonder that diabetics among others are honestly confused!

The term "lipid" as used in the United States includes neutral fat, fatty acids, steroids, waxes and phospholipids. Generally included in a discussion of lipids is cholesterol, which is found in animal fats and oils. Many persons who have elevated levels of cholesterol in the blood also have elevated levels of other blood lipids. In grossly uncontrolled diabetes, sometimes the levels of these lipids are several times higher than normal. With many such patients, the use of insulin and diet causes much improvement, and cholesterol levels, which have been as high as 2000 mg. per cent, have returned to normal (usually 150 to 250 mg. per cent) after proper treatment.

However, cholesterol itself normally has an important function in the body. It is formed in the liver and is so essential that the body manufactures its own if enough is not provided. Reduction of body weight in overweight persons often results in lowering blood cholesterol levels. The overweight diabetic also tends to have high triglyceride (other fatty acids) and uric acid levels.

If blood cholesterol levels are high, the physician will likely prescribe a modified diet, eliminating high-cholesterol foods such as egg yolks, kidney, oysters and lobster, as well as foods high in saturated fats including butter, whole milk, beef, lamb and pork. In general, the saturated fats are animal, and polyunsaturated fats are vegetable. Blood cholesterol levels that are too high may result in thickening of the inner linings of the blood vessels. The average American today consumes about 800 mg. of cholesterol a day. Some of the high-cholesterol foods are shown in Table 5.

Although scientists disagree about the effects of cholesterol and some feel that the anticholesterol data are not completely proven, most physicians believe that the proportion of polyunsaturated fat to saturated fat is probably important. It has been estimated that the average American diet has a ratio of polyunsaturated to saturated fat of about 0.3 to 1. Many physicians believe that the ratio should be at least 1 to 1.

Diet and Heart Disease.   Although statistical studies show a high association of elevated blood fats and cholesterol with increased cardiovascular disease, the question remains whether this is a coincidence or does indeed represent a

TABLE 5. Cholesterol Content of Some Foods

	Food	Cholesterol
Egg	Whole	275 mg.
	Yolk	275 mg.
	White	0 mg.
Meat	Beef	21 mg./ounce
	Brain	606 mg./ounce
	Chicken	18 mg./ounce
	Kidney	114 mg./ounce
	Lamb	21 mg./ounce
	Liver	91 mg./ounce
	Pork	21 mg./ounce
	Sweetbreads	132 mg./ounce
	Veal	27 mg./ounce
Dairy Foods	Butter	13 mg./tsp.
	Cottage cheese	4 mg./ounce
	Cream cheese	18 mg./ounce
	Ice cream	30 mg./half cup
	Skim milk	3 mg./half cup
	Whole milk	13 mg./half cup

cause-and-effect relationship. The data are not conclusive. For example, although the Japanese have been increasingly eating fatty foods and dairy products since 1955, the death rate due to heart attacks has actually decreased. An oft-quoted Harvard Medical School study observed 600 Irishmen who lived in Boston, matching them in each case with brothers who had remained in Ireland. Although those in Ireland ate 500 more calories daily and nearly twice as much butter and eggs as their brothers in the United States, they had lower cholesterol levels and less high blood pressure and weighed less than their brothers in Boston. Furthermore, people in Great Britain and Sweden eat almost the same amount of fat with the same ratio of fatty acids as do people in the United States. However, the death rate from coronary heart disease in the United States is three times higher than that of Sweden and twice as high as Great Britain's. The problem is further complicated by the fact that there are two types of cholesterol, high-density (HDL) and low-density lipoproteins (LDL). The LDL type causes problems, while the HDL type apparently carries much less risk.

Meanwhile, what should the person with diabetes do? His

physician will probably prescribe a diet lower in fat in general and may substitute foods containing polyunsaturated fat for those with animal fat. This can be done by using very lean cuts of meat and more poultry and fish, avoiding excessive use of eggs and, for adults, drinking fat-free milk. Many physicians recommend the use of margarines made from 100% corn oil in place of butter. Of course, the body weight should be reduced to normal or slightly lower. Remember, however, that polyunsaturated and animal fats both contain nine calories per gram. Diets too high in carbohydrate can also increase the amounts of blood triglycerides because the body manages to convert the excess glucose to fatty acids. Exercise and the discontinuance of cigarette smoking are other factors said to be helpful in lowering blood fat levels. In addition, certain medications have been useful in reducing high triglycerides.

coffee, tea or milk

No calorie difference exists between coffee and tea; if drunk plain, neither has calories. Large amounts of coffee or tea can stimulate the nervous system and cause sleeplessness. Milk, known as "the perfect food" because it is easily available and contains carbohydrate, protein and fat, is a good form of nutrition for babies, growing youngsters and some adults. Whole milk contains about 20 calories per ounce, which may be more than overweight adults need. Milk with fat removed (skim milk, nonfat milk) has only 10 calories per ounce.

eating while traveling

Suggestions about traveling with diabetes are discussed further in Chapter 11. However, travel is not the chore that it used to be. Of course, the diabetic should follow the usual routine with regard to meal and snack times as closely as possible. Ordinarily, in those parts of the world frequently visited, he should encounter little difficulty with eating. It might be well to keep fresh fruit, such as an orange or two or a small apple, in the hotel room or handbag in case meals are delayed. It is also important to check the customary meal hours in various countries; in some areas, the evening meal is served very much later than in the United States.

the vitamin culture

Americans are faddists by nature. In recent years, everyone has been vitamin-conscious. Vitamins are mysterious entities, most obvious when they are inadequate in the diet. The textbooks introduce the subject with, "A vitamin may be broadly defined as a substance that is essential for the maintenance of normal metabolic functions but which is not synthesized in the body and, therefore, must be furnished from an exogenous (outside) source." As shown in Table 6, vitamins do perform necessary functions. However, in recent years, many wild claims have been made for massive vitamin doses that are largely unsupported by objective evidence. Indeed, probably no group of drugs has been as misused as have vitamins. Although daily *minimum* allowances are known, optimal or ideal amounts are uncertain.

There are two types of vitamins: water-soluble vitamins, such as those in the B complex and vitamin C, and fat-soluble vitamins, A, D, and K. Other less understood compounds exist, such as vitamin P, found in citrus fruit peelings and alleged to prevent increased permeability of blood vessel walls.

While poor eating habits and some ethnic dietary customs may result in poor nutrition and inadequate vitamin intake, it is difficult to avoid vitamins. They are found in most foods, obviously more in some than in others.

Vitamin A is found in butter, milk, cheese, liver and many vegetables, especially the yellow vegetables such as carrots. Deficiency may impair growth and causes certain disorders of vision, the commonest of which is "night blindness." *Vitamin B* has been isolated into numerous components, some of which are useful in maintaining optimal body tone and nerve nutrition. Vitamin B deficiency may result in neuropathy. Beri-beri is a result of insufficient B_1. Shortage of another vitamin B fraction causes pellagra, found especially in parts of the world where large amounts of corn are eaten along with a greatly imbalanced diet. Anemias can occur from a deficit of B_{12}, a vitamin found in leafy green vegetables, nuts, fruits, yeast, whole grain and liver. *Vitamin D* is the classic vitamin that ensures the development of strong teeth and bones. Rickets results from a lack of this vitamin, which is produced by the body by exposure to sunshine, has been added to milk and occurs in the traditional cod liver oils of childhood memory.

Vitamin K is also vital, and a deficit of this vitamin for any reason, including poor absorption, may produce bleeding due to failure of the blood to clot normally. This vitamin is found in the leaves of alfalfa and in many other plants and vegetables.

Persons with or without diabetes who use a well-planned diet do not require vitamin supplements, although the all-purpose polyvitamin is harmless, and it is difficult to argue with the improved subjective well-being many claim to experience with a daily vitamin supplement. Vitamin deficiencies usually should be treated with specific replacements. Supplemental vitamins may be useful and indeed necessary with extremely rigorous or imbalanced diets, in malnutrition and in special situations such as surgery.

Vitamin preparations now have a sales volume of about 350 million dollars yearly in the United States. Many are harmless, being readily destroyed or eliminated from the body. However, some vitamins in very large doses can be harmful. High doses of vitamin A taken for prolonged periods can be risky, particularly for pregnant women and their fetuses. In pregnant animals, huge doses of vitamin A produce central nervous system changes and anomalies in the offspring.

Vitamin D preparations must also be used with caution. Massive doses may produce calcifications in many parts of the body, including the kidneys. Other possible effects include convulsions, acute pancreatitis and bone depletion. Some people are sensitive to vitamin D and do not realize it.

The High Tide of Vitamin C. Vitamin C has an important and proven function; a lack of this vitamin causes scurvy, the scourge of seafarers in sailing vessel days. It is readily found in foods, especially in citrus fruits and juices, cabbage, green peppers and a host of other vegetables. However, recently a great controversy has concerned the use of massive doses of vitamin C for the alleged cure of many conditions but chiefly for prevention of colds. This theory was given impetus by the enthusiastic espousal of Dr. Linus Pauling, a respected two-time Nobel Prize winner, who has been quoted as saying that large doses of vitamin C (up to 10 grams a day) not only are harmless but greatly reduce the incidence of the common cold. He believes that the vitamin acts by synthesizing a substance called "interferon" which stops the cold virus from entering

TABLE 6. Vitamins

Vitamin	Sources	Daily Allowance*	Unit	Known Uses
A	whole milk, butter, fortified margerine, eggs, yellow vegetables, leafy green vegetables, liver	5000	I.U.	Promotes growth and development of bones and teeth; helps maintain vision in dim light; prevents dry, bumpy skin.
B_1 Thiamine	whole grain, enriched bread or cereals, yeast, liver, pork, fish, lean meat, poultry, milk	1.5	mg	Protects against beriberi, a deficiency disease common in the 19th century among those who lived on diets of refined or polished rice; useful in the metabolic breakdown of carbohydrates and for normal functioning of nervous system.
B_2 Riboflavin	milk, whole grain, enriched bread and cereals, liver, lean meat, eggs, leafy green vegetables	1.7	mg	Deficiency in diet causes young animals to grow and develop improperly; possible relationship to nutritional anemia.
B_6 Pyridoxine	lean meats, leafy green vegetables, whole grain cereals	2	mg	Causes poor function of nervous system—a rare deficiency.
B_{12} Cyanocobalamine	liver, kidney, fish, milk, foods of animal origin in general	6	μg	Inadequate B_{12} causes large red blood cell type of anemia. When the body doesn't absorb B_{12}, pernicious anemia may result.
Folic Acid	leafy green vegetables, liver	0.4	mg	Lack causes poor growth and development and certain types of anemia.
Pantothenic Acid	eggs, leafy green vegetables, nuts, liver, kidney	10	mg	Deficiency not known in man.

	Food sources	RDA*	Units	Description
Niacin	eggs, meat, liver, whole grain and enriched breads and cereals	20	mg	Adequate amounts prevent pellagra, early stages of muscle weakness, appetite loss and skin eruptions; later effects on nervous system.
Biotin	liver, kidney, eggs, leafy green vegetables	0.3	mg	Deficiency in man not seen but is involved in metabolic processes.
C	citrus fruits mostly; also other fruits, leafy green vegetables, potatoes	60	mg	Preventive against scurvy, formerly a disease of sea voyagers because of lack of fresh fruits; helps collagen develop (this material keeps cells in place); helps healing; decreases the possibility of some infections.
D	fortified milk, cod liver oil, egg yolk, tuna, salmon	400	I.U.	Necessary to provide normal development of bones and teeth; the need starts even before birth. Deficiency causes rickets. Some is present in skin and becomes active on exposure to the sun.
E	vegetable oils, whole grain cereals	30	I.U.	Not too much known about vitamin E. Has prevented sterility in rats and is present in many common foods, particularly wheat germ. Some possibility of relationship to polyunsaturated fatty acids.
K	leafy green vegetables			Helps blood to clot normally; known as anti-hemorrhage vitamin.

* Recommended daily allowance in adults and children age 4 or more. Pregnant or lactating women or infants and small children use different doses.
Measurement units: I.U. = International units; mg = milligrams; μg = micrograms

the cell. Many medical authorities question this alleged capacity of vitamin C, and although Dr. Pauling's approach may merit experimental study, it has yet to be verified. Some reports suggest that vitamin C may some day prove helpful in the cellular metabolism of diabetics, but this again has not been verified. Despite the foregoing, many persons claim that they "feel better and have fewer colds" when using vitamin C. Yet in locations where diets are naturally very high in this vitamin C, the number of colds does not appear to decrease. Vitamin C preparations are relatively inexpensive and generally harmless, but a well-balanced diet should replenish it. Large doses should be avoided by patients with a history of gout. In addition, ingestion of large doses of vitamin C may cause unreliable results in some of the dip and tape tests for urine glucose. This may pose a hazard for the diabetic, especially since both false positive and negative tests have been reported.

The Vitamin E Fad. Another preparation that is the darling of both vitamin addicts and sellers of health foods is vitamin E, also known as the anti-aging vitamin. A leading researcher was quoted as saying, "Vitamin E is one of those embarrassing vitamins that have been identified, isolated and synthesized by physiologists and biochemists and then handed to the medical profession with a suggestion that a use should be found for it, without any satisfactory evidence to show that human beings are ever deficient of it or even that it is a necessary nutrient for man." Its very nonspecificity has attracted legions of faddists who claim more cures than diseases needing cures. The claims are for every possible affliction, regardless of the body system or the dosage, and none has ever been proven by any adequate studies. Vitamin E is commonly found in foods and there appears to be no evidence of a deficiency in the population as a whole. The Canadian Dietary Standard states, "Evidence suggests that vitamin E is probably required by humans, but there is no evidence upon which a valid estimate of vitamin E requirement may be based." There is no evidence that supplements of vitamin E are necessary or especially helpful to diabetics, but they are probably harmless in ordinary doses.

minerals

Minerals are involved in many body functions. Copper and iron are necessary for blood building. Sodium, chloride and potassium are electrolyte constituents of the blood and body cells. Manganese and zinc as well as other of the so-called "trace" elements are widely found in foods and almost no one needs to take supplemental amounts. When, as a result of certain diseases, patients have too little, then sodium, potassium or chloride can readily be given as needed.

dietetic foods and food fads

Special foods are not necessary for diabetics, who are often confused by the word "dietetic." *Dietetic* does not mean *diabetic*. *Dietetic* food can denote a decrease in calories or some other modification of contents. The calories and/or the carbohydrate content may still exceed acceptable limits for diabetics (see Appendix 5).

During recent hospital rounds, a patient with diabetes proudly pointed to a box of "diabetic chocolates" which had been given to him. Knowing the manufacturer's reputation for elegant chocolates, the dietitian searched and found minute letters on the side of the box that stated that each chocolate had "only 60 calories" (possibly their regular chocolates contained 130 calories each). The patient had been happily nibbling in the false belief that they were "diabetic." This is the hazard of alleged dietetic foods. They may have *fewer* calories, but fewer than what? If a person wishes to indulge and clearly knows the contents of the food in carbohydrate value and calories, and if these levels can be fitted into the framework of the diet, the food may be permissible. However, it is confusing when labels indicate the presence of "dextrins," "disaccharides" or words ending in "-tol" and "-ose." These words generally mean some type of sugar. In addition, the cost of such foods is much higher than that of regular foods.

Labels—Information and Confusion.   One encounters pitfalls in trying to track through the jungle of labels. Labels are difficult to read and hard to understand. The words do not always mean what they appear to say, reminiscent of the declaration of Humpty-Dumpty who stated that when *he* used a word, the word meant exactly what *he* intended it to mean. Particularly in so-called dietetic foods, the label should state what is in the package, how it has been processed and the contents. In addition to vague items such as "0.1% sodium benzoate as a preservative," the label might state that the product contains 5000 times more vitamin D than some other food. Labels should mention the amounts of carbohydrate, protein and fat. However, these should be given in relationship to an individual serving and not merely as percentages of the net weight of the whole package. Many people do not understand even simple foods such as "buttermilk" (milk from which the cream has been removed in order to make butter). Cocoa is chocolate from which the fat has been removed. Vegetable margarine has the same amount of fat and calories as butter but contains no animal fat, and so on. With new federal requirements, labels will be much clearer and useful to consumers, diabetics included. There will be an insistence on labelling food contents as well as calories per serving and the percentage of the recommended daily allowance of each item. The labelling of fat content will give the amounts of polyunsaturated and saturated fats. Further restrictions will establish definite standards for dietetic and special foods.

The Vegetarian Diet and Organic Foods. Many people use a largely or completely vegetarian diet. Some simply eat no meat while others avoid not only meat but also fowl, eggs, milk and other dairy products. With a completely vegetarian diet that excludes even milk and milk products, essential amino acids are difficult to obtain. At present, no hard evidence exists that a completely vegetarian diet protects its users from degenerative complications. However, with culinary skill, one can devise a healthful and enjoyable meatless diet.

The Zen Macrobiotic and Other Single Food Diets. Some of these diets are comprised completely of cereals. Severe nutritional deficiencies have been reported in persons who follow such regimens for significant periods of time.

Organic Diets. "Organic" foods are grown with the aid of fertilizers of animal or vegetable origin, and are fancied by many people who will eat nothing but such foods. We have no good evidence that foods grown in this manner make much difference nutritionally, although much is not yet known about the long-term effects of chemical fertilizers and additives. The effects of these food habits are the same for the diabetic as for the nondiabetic.

food additives

In recent years, volumes have been written about food additives, which came into common use when foods were processed and shipped thousands of miles for storage or sale. The most common additive is sodium chloride or table salt, some of which is essential to everyone. Sodium chloride is usually harmless to diabetics unless they have a heart or kidney condition or high blood pressure, which requires salt restriction. Another common additive is monosodium glutamate. In susceptible persons, this agent may cause an acute illness characterized by headache, weakness and gastrointestinal distress.

Surprisingly, after salt, sucrose (ordinary cane sugar) is one of the most common food additives, which may provide one reason for the steady increase in sugar consumption. It is also another reason why diabetics should read labels carefully.

A whole group of substances is known as GRAS (meaning "Generally Recognized as Safe" for their intended use). These include coloring agents, curing and pickling agents, drying agents, enzymes, flavor enhancers, processing aids, and non-nutrient sweeteners. A coloring agent known as "red dye" was removed from the market in 1976 because of potentially harmful effects. However, additives are probably here to stay because without them, it would not be possible to package, ship, store or even process foods suited to modern convenience requirements. Except for salt and sugar, the effects of additives are the same for diabetics and nondiabetics.

other sugars

It is easy to be confused when certain sugars such as fructose are listed as "good for diabetics" or as "dietetic" sugars. Because of special features in the metabolism of these sugars, it was once thought that they would be utilized in spite of insufficient insulin. In general, the ability of the liver to use glucose is decreased in diabetics, but the ability to utilize fructose proceeds at a normal rate. Fructose does not require the presence of insulin to be metabolized by the body, and it is absorbed rapidly by both diabetics and nondiabetics. However, fructose is also stored rapidly as glycogen, which is broken down into glucose when the body requires fuel for energy. Unless insulin is available, the ingestion of fructose ultimately results in high levels of blood sugar. Therefore, while fructose differs from glucose in its early use, its addition to foods does not provide any practical help to the diabetic. Any advantages to be gained lie in its use in research.

Sorbitol and mannitol are "sugar alcohols." Although they are carbohydrate in nature, they are absorbed slowly from the intestine. However, they are converted to glucose in the body. Because sorbitol in particular is used widely in commercially prepared foods, one should read the labels of "dietetic" foods. The diabetic can tolerate small amounts of sorbitol and mannitol better than sugar, but should avoid eating larger amounts, not only because of the effect on diabetes, but because these chemicals tend to cause diarrhea.

gourmet eating

Unquestionably, if a person wishes to devote the time and effort needed for the preparation of elegant recipes, with sufficient knowledge even the diabetic can eat meals that might be classified as gourmet. Indeed, one can prepare elaborate low-calorie foods for the obese as well as the diabetic. However, many people have neither the knowledge nor the motivation to make a hobby of exquisite dining and prefer simple foods, simply prepared. For those who may be interested, the gustatory rewards can be great.

special food and drinks for athletes

Along with the boom in sports, interest has risen in special liquid supplements for athletes and others who exercise strenuously. The replacement of fluid and salts in such persons is important because sweating can deplete body electrolytes (e.g., sodium, potassium) and lead to changes in the blood chemistry. Severe depletion may cause collapse. In hot weather and under conditions of extreme activity, the fluid and actual weight loss can be considerable. Milk can replace many of the constituents, but it does not necessarily quench the thirst and it contains protein and fat which are slow to digest during strenuous exercise. Ginger ale and cola beverages can be used; they have a large amount of carbohydrate (about 80 to 110 calories in 8 ounces). Cola drinks contain a slight amount of caffeine which encourages further sweating. Special drinks called "-ades" (such as Gatorade) have been devised which contain all the necessary electrolytes as well as carbohydrate and fluid. Since football players on a hot day may lose about 10 calories a minute, a 90-minute session would cost about 900 calories.

The so-called -ades may be useful for replacing body fluids and electrolytes in a hurry, but only under unusual circumstances and strictly for athletes. These products are not ordinarily intended for diabetics.

the economics of diet

Food costs are increasing worldwide. Even in places where food is relatively inexpensive, it costs more than before, and the economics of more people sharing the same resources on earth means that food costs will continue to rise in the future. This causes problems for diabetics because carbohydrates are the least expensive foods; proteins and fats cost much more. Meat or its substitutes are vital to body growth and maintenance. However, as the increasing world population competes for protein, getting a balanced diet becomes increasingly difficult. Fortunately there is little nutritional difference between expensive meats and lower cost cuts, and other protein foods, such as beans, can substitute for meat. Even now, the thrifty shopper can obtain 20 grams of protein (nearly one-third of the daily adult requirement) from other sources for one-tenth the price of the same amount of protein in the form of steak. Of course, soybeans will increase in price, but steak costs will increase faster. Interestingly, many nutritionists believe that Americans eat too much meat; they suggest that protein be obtained from more economical sources, such as poultry, fish, eggs, cheese, peanut butter and some grains. Regardless of the grade, all eggs have the same nutritional content. Grade B eggs are not as delicate and may not have as firm a yolk as Grade A eggs, but they have the same amounts of protein and fat. Day-old bread is every bit as nutritious as fresh bread. The following list compares sources of protein; the most expensive per unit appears at the top of the list and the least expensive at the bottom.

> Loin lamb chops
> Bacon
> Sirloin steak
> Pork loin roast
> Frozen fish fillets
> Turkey
> American cheese
> Canned tuna
> Large eggs
> Dried beans

A good means of obtaining protein is to use more fish and seafood. Pound for pound, fish provides as much protein as beef with only half the calories. Also, the fats are probably less harmful. Thus, while eating may be more expensive than formerly, one can still obtain a balanced diet at a lower cost by using ingenuity in the choice of foods.

the "new" high-carbohydrate diet

Much interest has been manifested concerning a "new" high-carbohydrate diet for diabetics. A study of persons with mild diabetes in a Veterans Administration Hospital reported improved glucose tolerance with high carbohydrate feeding. With the use of insulin, more generous portions of carbohydrate have become increasingly common in diabetic diets. A committee of the American Diabetes Association recently stated, "There no longer appears to be any need to restrict disproportionately the intake of carbohydrate in the diet of most diabetic patients." Note the word "disproportionately." The committee further pointed out that "the physician or dietitian should never forget that careful control of the food the diabetic eats is still the basic treatment of mild and moderately severe cases of diabetes of the maturity-onset type." The fact is that when carbohydrates are used or adequately stored, they pose no problem. However, no one suggests that a diet of straight sugar or sweets or large amounts of starch-rich foods be permitted for those who promptly lose much of the carbohydrate they have eaten in the urine. Although diet prescriptions may vary with different physicians and institutions, the differences are more apparent than real. Few, if any, permit diabetics to eat all they want of everything. With this "new" diet concept, *calorie control is not relaxed* and most diabetics, particularly those who require insulin, still are not free to choose anything they may want. The goal remains the avoidance of those amounts and types of carbohydrate that result in greatly elevated blood sugar levels and much loss of sugar in the urine while maintaining a balanced diet that avoids the two extremes of feast and famine.

summary

In summary, diet is not merely important but vital for most people, and particularly so for diabetics. Diets of one type or another are being used increasingly by much of the population, whether to lose weight or to treat hypertension, heart disease, ulcer and a myriad of other conditions. The dieter is no longer unique. Diabetic diets have improved. With ingenuity and effort, those with diabetes can eat adequately and well and many have even learned to prepare elegant meals. Some people find any type of restriction or change distasteful, and they are not likely to be enthusiastic about diet either. Once diabetics recognize that the purpose of a diet is not to deny them food, but to enable them to choose foods they like that will remain with them, they will find, as many already have, that the sacrifices are small compared to the benefits gained.

4

Insulin

4

Few developments in medicine have so changed the course of a disease and given life to so many as the advent of insulin. After Banting and Best developed insulin in 1921 and the first reports came from Toronto, Dr. Elliott P. Joslin said, "With the bright news from Toronto, a hope for life." The first insulin was known as "isletin" because of its origin in the islets of Langerhans of the pancreas. Later the term "insulin" was adopted because it had been used by earlier investigators. This hormone, a protein made up of two connected chains of amino acids, cannot be taken by mouth because it is digested by the action of the enzymes in the stomach and intestines. Also, no chain of amino acids can be absorbed through the intestinal wall without losing its configuration. The amino acids of each species of animal occurs in a special sequence, almost like a fingerprint. Strangely, the insulin most like that of a human is from the pig; only the end amino acid is different. Insulin from almost any animal is effective in humans, but the varying arrangements of the amino acids may be a cause of excessive antibody production, which tends to make insulin less effective.

In the United States and throughout the world, most of the insulin comes from the pancreases of cattle and pigs. In countries where large numbers of sheep are used for food, insulin can be made from sheep pancreas. Useful insulin has been made from whales and, in Japan, from tuna fish or indeed nearly any animal. However, the world population increases and so do the numbers of diabetics. The demands for insulin grow. Pancreases for insulin are increasingly prized. Moreover, some people are trying to persuade the populations of the world to eat less meat in order to make more grain available to feed more people. If the use of cattle for meat decreases and the number of diabetics around the world increases, measures must be taken to ensure that every available pancreas is utilized; indeed, these glands are now widely sought in even the most undeveloped parts of the world.

As marketed, insulin is quite stable. Even after a year at room temperature, only a small percentage of its potency is lost. However, any reserve supply of insulin should be refrigerated (40° F). At constant high temperatures (greater than 86° F) the loss of strength is only 2.3% in two months; after constant high heat (104° F), about 10% of strength is lost.

The normal fasting blood level of insulin in humans varies from 1 to 30 microunits in 1 cc. (1 milliliter) of blood. A microunit is 1/1,000,000 of a unit of insulin. Obviously, even in nondiabetic persons, the amount of insulin actually circulating in the blood at one time is very small. This amount increases after each meal and returns to the normal fasting level in about three hours. In normal persons, insulin is supplied in amounts appropriate to the needs of the moment.

characteristics of insulin

The diabetic must know the characteristics of insulin, the times of its greatest activity (peak) and duration of action (Table 7). Symptoms of low blood sugar levels, which range from simply annoying to acutely distressing, may result from too much insulin. With this knowledge, the insulin dose can often be adjusted by doing urine tests for sugar at various times of the day.

Because plain insulin (known also as regular or crystalline insulin in the United States and as Toronto insulin in Canada) in solution has a short period of action in the body, it would have to be used three, four or more times daily to be ideally effective during the 24-hour period. This fast-acting, short-duration insulin was the only kind available for 15 years after the discovery of insulin. Many diabetic patients required four or even five injections daily for good control. A few such patients never discontinued this program and have continued to take insulin several times a day through all these years. Some have done extremely well, probably because this method of delivery most nearly imitates normal pancreatic function.

Types of Insulin. In order to decrease the number of required daily injections, certain materials have been added to

TABLE 7. Characteristics of Insulin
A. Summary of Commonly Used Insulin Preparations

Description	Regular	NPH	Lente	Protamine Zinc
Concentration (units per cc or ml)	40, 80, 100	40, 80, 100	40, 80, 100	40, 80, 100
Modifying agent (amount per 100 units)	None	Protamine, 0.3 to 0.6 mg	None (acetate buffer)	Protamine, 1.0 to 1.5 mg
Proportion of bound insulin	None	67%	None	100%
Zinc (amount per 100 units)	None	0.016 to 0.04 mg.	0.2 to 0.25 mg.	0.2 to 0.25 mg
Route of administration	Intravenous or subcutaneous	Subcutaneous	Subcutaneous	Subcutaneous
Can be mixed with regular insulin?	—	Yes	Yes	Yes, but not usually done

B. Action of Commonly Used Insulins

Type of Insulin & Appearance	Onset of Action (in hours)	Peak of Action (in hours)	Duration of Action (in hours)
SHORT-ACTING (RAPID)			
Crystalline or Regular: clear	1	2–4	6–8
Semilente: cloudy	1½–2	4–7	12–16
INTERMEDIATE (SLOW)			
Globin: clear	2–4	10–14	14–22
NPH (Isophane):* cloudy	1–2	10–16	18–30
Lente:* cloudy	1–2	10–16	18–30
PROLONGED (VERY SLOW)			
Protamine Zinc: cloudy when shaken	6–8	14–24	24–36
Ultralente: cloudy or milky after shaking	5–8	20–26	36 or longer

*NPH and Lente insulins are generally considered to be interchangeable.

insulin to prolong its action. Adding protamine, a simple protein, and zinc in a certain concentration resulted in the formulation of protamine zinc insulin in 1935. This insulin usually lasts somewhat longer than 24 hours. Later, this preparation was modified by decreasing the amount of protamine and changing the zinc concentration, resulting in isophane or NPH insulin in 1950 (NPH means neutral protamine Hagedorn, honoring the developer of this intermediate-acting insulin). Later modifications produced the Lente family of insulin zinc suspensions: Lente, Semilente and Ultralente. Lente is an intermediate-acting insulin that resembles NPH in its effect; in fact, one can usually use these two preparations interchangeably. Semilente is an insulin of short duration (though somewhat longer than regular insulin). Ultralente has a prolonged duration (roughly comparable to protamine zinc insulin). Throughout the world, these are the most commonly used types of insulin. Another type, still used in some parts of the world but decreasingly in the United States, is globin insulin. The action of globin insulin lasts longer than regular insulin but shorter than the intermediate insulins.

Table 7 also shows the various types of insulin available, which are normally prepared from a mixture of insulin crystals extracted from both beef and pork pancreas. The mixture is roughly 70% beef and 30% pork, although these proportions may vary with the availability of pancreases. Eli Lilly and Co. manufactures regular and modified insulins, NPH, protamine zinc, and Lente, Semilente and Ultralente in U-40, U-80, and U-100 strengths. The brand name for insulin produced by Lilly is Iletin. Although this company no longer makes pure pork or pure beef insulin in the U-40 strength, these preparations are available in the U-100 strength.

E.R. Squibb and Sons manufacture regular, globin, NPH, protamine zinc, and Lente, Semilente, and Ultralente insulins in the U-40, U-80, and U-100 strengths. The three Lente-type insulins are prepared only from beef pancreases; the other insulins are a mixture of beef and pork. Regular insulin in the U-100 strength contains more pork than beef insulin; in all other insulins, beef is the predominant source.

The Insulin Unit.   Insulin is measured in units. This appears on the label as "U," which means "clinical unit." A *unit* is always constant because it measures a specific amount of activity. The unit is the same for *every* insulin. This international standard or measurement is consistent throughout the world. Insulin is a powerful substance, because a single unit may remove an amount of sugar many times its own weight from the bloodstream.

One unit of U-40 insulin is exactly the same and performs the same work as 1 unit of U-80, 1 unit of U-100 or any other strength of insulin. The only difference is the matter of dilution; U-40 has twice as much water mixed with a given amount of insulin as does U-80. One unit is still exactly 1 unit whether it is concentrated as U-40, U-80, U-100 or even U-500. The numbers only tell the total number of units of insulin that are dissolved in 1 milliliter (1 cubic centimeter or $\frac{1}{30}$ of an ounce). Usually this is one syringeful. In the past, U-40 insulin was used by those taking small amounts because it is easier to measure in the usual syringe. This problem will soon disappear because eventually all patients will be using U-100 insulin only. It is important to remember that, whatever strength of insulin is used, *the patient must use the same type of insulin syringe (U-40, U-80, U-100) as the strength of the insulin used.*

Eventually, only U-100 insulin will be available. Meanwhile, since other strengths of insulin are still available, the only real protection against inaccurate dosage is to READ THE LABEL and BE CERTAIN YOUR INSULIN STRENGTH AND SYRINGE MARKINGS ARE THE SAME.

Labels and Bottle Shapes. Various codes of label colors and bottle shapes have been used to help patients identify the different strengths of insulin. However, many believe that the use of colored labels (not always uniform) to specify strengths is not protective because many users cannot distinguish colors well. *The only real protection is to read the label.* Besides, there are not enough useful colors to distinguish the differences in insulins. Eventually, only insulins of U-100 strength plan to be marketed, which is now done in Canada. Varieties of U-100 insulin are marketed in round bottles with white labels that have black printing.

While various strengths are still available, U-80 insulin has green labels and U-40 has red. (U-80 Lente has a lavender label.) Round bottles are used to denote both regular (short-acting) and protamine zinc (very long-acting) types of insulin, in both U-40 and U-80 strengths. Semilente (short), Lente (intermediate) and Ultralente (long-acting) insulins are marketed in six-sided "shoulder" bottles.

The clearness of the insulin also provides a good identifying feature. Regular insulin is always clear, even after being shaken; all modified insulins (NPH, Lente and protamine zinc) look cloudy or milky after being shaken gently. Globin insulin is always clear.

The Emergency Insulin.   For emergencies, regular (also known as crystalline, clear, rapid, fast-acting) is the insulin of choice. This basic insulin is effective almost at once after injection and has a short duration. Every patient with diabetes should have a bottle of regular insulin on hand for emergencies whether they need it each day or not. It will retain potency indefinitely if kept in the refrigerator.

Storage.   Storing insulin poses no problem. Always have at least one or two extra bottles on hand. Insulin should be stored in the refrigerator at about 40° F, but *not* in the freezing compartment. Frozen insulin loses its potency.

As pointed out previously, the bottle in current use may be kept at room temperature, as some patients may find cold insulin unpleasant when injected. If extremes of temperature are avoided, insulin can be kept at room temperature for months without having any significant loss in strength. The expiration date on every bottle of insulin has a large safety margin. This is a minimum date before which there is absolutely no question about the potency of the insulin. After the expiration date, the insulin may start losing strength.

Discard any bottle of regular insulin that may be cloudy or discolored. This type of insulin should always be clear. Patients sometimes claim that the insulin loses potency as the bottle is almost used up. This might be due to inadvertent freezing of the insulin, or to some contamination of the insulin. The safest step is to discard such insulin.

Insulins Abroad.   Patients sometimes worry about obtaining insulin when traveling in foreign countries. The preparation of insulin is standardized throughout the world, regardless of the manufacturer, so that units are the same (although in some areas only U-40 insulin may be available). In many parts of the world, American-manufactured insulins are available. See Appendix 6 for names of insulin preparations found elsewhere in the world and their relationship to preparations commonly used here.

Patients sometimes ask whether a "kosher" insulin is available. None is available in this country, although insulin derived from pure beef extracts can be obtained by those who might be concerned about the animal origin of their insulin. However, rabbinical decisions have stated that any medicine necessary for life, such as insulin, can be used regardless of the source.

"Single-Peak" and "Monocomponent" Insulins. Until recently, insulin preparations were about 93% pure. The "impurities" were not contaminants, but other chemicals including insulin-like substances and glucagon that remained in the insulin after processing. Modern techniques have improved the product so that now insulin is almost 99% pure. "Single-peak" insulin is so named because electrochemical studies show "one peak" on a tracing, i.e., it is composed of mostly one substance. It was hoped that this purer insulin would cause less immunologic resistance with less antibody formation. Some tests have shown that its use may prevent or correct fat atrophy beneath the skin at sites of insulin injection. *Since 1972 all insulin sold in the United States has been of this single-peak type.* Eli Lilly and Company uses the designation "single-peak" for its insulins; E.R. Squibb and Sons uses the designation "high purity" or "single-peak quality."

"Monocomponent" insulin is different. This is the purest insulin available and has only *one* component. It is not sold in this country because of the difficulty of large-scale manufacturing.

syringes for insulin

Many types of syringes are available for use with insulin, which may be confusing. Those most commonly used and approved by the American Diabetes Association have only one

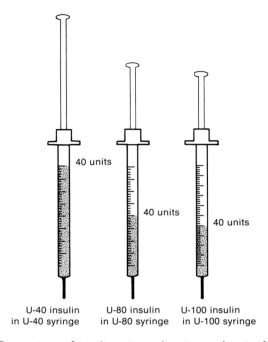

FIG. 17. Comparison of insulin units and syringes. A unit of insulin is still a unit regardless which type of insulin is used, *if* the correct syringe is used. Each syringe contains 40 units, but the amounts of insulin in the syringes are progressively smaller. This is because U-80 insulin is more concentrated than U-40 insulin, and U-100 insulin is more concentrated than U-80 or U-40 insulin. (Although the U-100 syringe appears to be about the same size, the barrel is more slender than the other syringes, which makes reading the scale easier.) When patients change to the new U-100 insulin, the same dose in units will be used, even though the liquid volume will be less.

type of scale on each syringe with the numbers marked in red for U-40 insulin or green for the U-80, just like the labels on the bottles. Figure 17 shows these syringes. A longer-barrel 2-cc syringe, graduated for U-80 insulin, holds 160 units; this is used by the few patients who use more than 80 units in a single injection. Syringes made by different manufacturers come in different thicknesses and lengths. Some are short and stubby and fit into travel kits. In any event, the syringe must be clearly marked for U-40, U-80 or U-100 insulin. Avoid syringes that have both U-40 and U-80 markings. This problem will disappear when only U-100 insulin is available. U-100 syringes are available in the following sizes: 50 units, 100 units (1 cc), and 200 units (2 cc).

People are concerned about the "dead space" that occurs between the end of the plunger and the tip of the syringe, where the needle attaches to the syringe. Some small amount of insulin may be trapped here and not be injected. Usually, so few units are involved that this does not make much difference. However, it may be significant with the use of U-100 insulin, or when the insulin dosage requires that a small dose of regular insulin be drawn into the syringe first, followed by a dose of NPH or Lente insulin. Some companies now manufacture syringes that have no "dead space." When purchasing syringes, diabetics should look for types that have the least distance remaining at the end of the syringe when the plunger is pushed down. As U-100 insulin becomes the standard insulin and greater emphasis is placed on disposable needle-syringe combinations, newer and improved types of syringes will have less dead space.

It cannot be emphasized sufficiently that 1 unit of insulin is exactly the same regardless of the strength. If a person injects 20 units of U-40, U-80 or U-100 insulin, the dose is exactly 20 units *if the syringe matches the insulin.* The difference is in concentration. If two persons each weigh 150 pounds, and one person is five feet tall while the other is six feet tall, they still both weigh 150 pounds each. The shorter man is a more concentrated package. In one study, 58% of all diabetic insulin errors were due to confusion about units.

U-100 Insulin. Conversion of all people who require insulin to the use of U-100 insulin is long overdue. It is a logical step and will simplify matters. Not only is there less chance for error, but because the insulin dose is delivered in a smaller volume, it should be less painful to inject. Also, a bottle of U-100 insulin lasts longer, simplifying storage. For those who require very small insulin doses, a U-100 syringe with a 50-unit capacity is available. This has graduations large enough that even 1 or 2 units can be measured readily. It is wise for all diabetics to convert to the new strength as soon as practicable. Changing over is easy. The same number of units are used, but the syringe units must match the insulin units.

ADVANTAGES OF U-100 INSULIN:

1. less chance of dosage error
2. smaller volume to be injected
3. more refined, purer insulin
4. more units per bottle (1,000), which means you can buy supplies less often and have to store fewer bottles
5. per unit cost, about the same as other strengths

Needles and Disposable Supplies. Hypodermic needles for insulin injection can vary in length from $\frac{3}{8}$ to $\frac{5}{8}$ of an inch. They also come in different gauges; 25 or 26 gauge is usually recommended. The needle gauge number indicates the thickness of the needle. The lower the number, the thicker the needle. For example, a 16-gauge needle would be wide; a 26-gauge needle would be very thin. The thinner the needle with a sharp point, the less the pain from injection. Stainless steel needles may be used over and over again, provided they are sterilized after each usage. They may be sharpened on a stone and used for many months. Because all reusable needles eventually bend, break or become dull, patients should have extras available.

Many patients now use disposable syringes and needles. These syringes are made of plastic and cannot be resterilized by boiling. The needles are made of a much softer metal than stainless steel and cannot be resharpened. Disposable syringes and needles are intended to be used for one injection only and then thrown away. Their long-term cost is higher than that for glass syringes and steel needles, but they are convenient for travel.

Reusable syringes and needles can be kept in alcohol between injections. Before filling the syringe with insulin, the alcohol must be expelled by pushing the plunger in and out a few times. Reusable syringes and steel needles should be sterilized by boiling approximately once weekly. Some patients combine both methods by using a glass syringe with disposable needles that can be changed daily.

how to inject insulin

This is the most important technique that diabetics must learn. Even those diabetics who use oral compounds or diet alone to control their disease may have to learn how to inject insulin because a time may come when they will need it. The most important facts are: (1) applying proper technique for injection, (2) choosing the right injection site and (3) having a schedule for rotating these sites. The following steps should be taken (*Fig. 18*):

1. Thoroughly but gently mix the insulin by upending the bottle and rolling it between the palms (*Fig. 18A*). Shaking the bottle creates bubbles. Wipe the insulin bottle top with 70% alcohol.

2. Draw air into the insulin syringe in the same amount as the insulin to be withdrawn (*Fig. 18B*). If 10 units are to be removed, leave 10 units of air in the syringe.

3. Insert the needle in the bottle, and push the plunger down (*Fig. 18C*).

4. Invert the bottle and draw more insulin into the syringe than needed. Push the plunger up, expelling the insulin and air bubbles. Do this several times to get rid of all air bubbles in the syringe (*Fig. 18D*).

5. Pull the plunger down slowly to the right amount of insulin (*Fig. 18E*).

6. Holding the syringe at an angle to the skin (15 to 20 degrees from the straight up-and-down), plunge the needle into the site that has been prepared by cleaning with alcohol (*Fig. 18F*). Push the plunger down all the way.

7. Quickly withdraw the needle, wipe with alcohol and gently rub the area of injection.

Keep in mind the following points while injecting insulin. It is best to grasp some tissue firmly between the thumb and one finger of one hand, holding the syringe in the other hand. Grasp a large amount of skin and tissue beneath the skin, although not too tightly, so that injection well beneath the surface of the skin is possible. Just before pushing the plunger to inject the insulin into the tissue, stop a second and gently pull the plunger up. A little blood will appear at the tip of the syringe if the needle is in a vein or small blood vessel. This is a signal to remove the needle and inject into a new place.

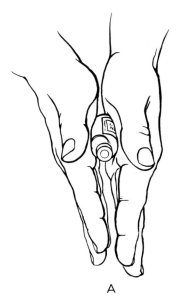

A

FIG. 18. A. The technique of injecting insulin accurately must be mastered by everyone who uses insulin. Slight errors can be serious. Begin by turning the bottle of insulin upside down and rolling it between the palms. The purpose of this step is to mix the insulin thoroughly.

FIG. 18. B. Next, carefully wipe off the top of the bottle with alcohol-soaked cotton. The next step is vital. Draw air into the syringe in the same amount *as the insulin dose* to be taken. In other words, if you need 20 units of insulin, you fill the syringe with 20 units of air, which is left in the syringe temporarily. The reason for this is that a vacuum exists in the insulin bottle, and in order to remove the insulin, you must first inject the same amount of air.

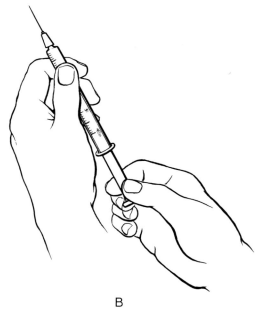

B

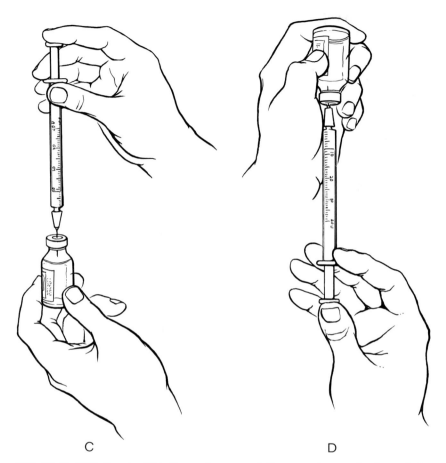

C   D

FIG. 18. C. With the air still in the syringe, carefully insert the needle through the diaphragm top into the bottle. Push the plunger down. D. Turn the bottle upside down and pull back the plunger to a point considerably past the amount of insulin needed. Push the insulin and air back into the bottle several times. The purpose of this step is to push all of the air bubbles back into the bottle of insulin.

Injecting insulin into a blood vessel poses no real danger, but bleeding and discoloration of the skin may occur when the needle is finally removed.

Don't be disturbed if a small amount of blood appears after withdrawing the needle. Simply press the spot gently and briefly with cotton soaked with alcohol. It is very important to

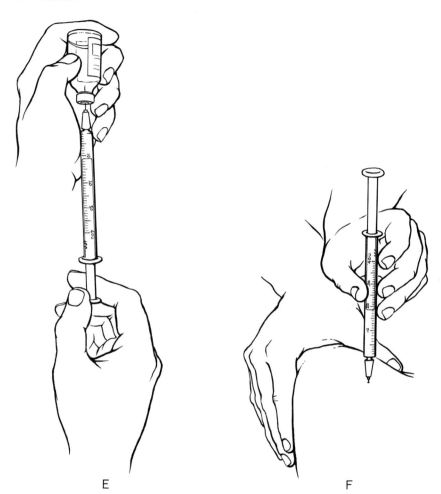

E   F

FIG. 18. E. Now that all the air bubbles are out of the syringe, carefully pull the plunger down to the correct amount of insulin. F. The syringe now has the precise amount of insulin required. Wipe the spot to be injected with cotton and alcohol, and pinch the skin. Holding the syringe like a pencil, push the needle straight into the skin and push the plunger down. Release the pinched skin, press the cotton ball next to the needle, and pull out.

keep a clean technique to avoid local infection. Infections and boils can occur when people are careless about injections.

How deep should the injection go? New diabetics are terrified, being certain that they will pierce some vital organ. This is almost impossible considering the short length of the needle used.

Removing Bubbles.

Patients worry about the tiny bubbles that sometimes appear in the syringe before giving insulin. To avoid bubbles, do not shake the insulin bottle too vigorously, but rather roll it gently between the palms of the hands for mixing. Then, after the insulin is in the syringe, hold the syringe vertically, tip up, and draw back a bit to unite all the bubbles into one big one. Then slowly push the air and bubbles out. However, do not worry if several bubbles still remain, because much greater amounts of air are necessary to do any damage to the patient and even then, the air would have to be put directly into a vein. The disadvantage of having any small bubbles in the insulin syringe is only that air displaces a certain amount of insulin so that the full dosage will not be given. Any error is likely to be small and insignificant.

Automatic and Jet Injectors.

Some diabetics, squeamish about injecting themselves directly, use a small automatic injector to insert the needle beneath the skin. This may be satisfactory if the injector is simple enough. The syringe is filled with insulin as usual and then the injector is spring-cocked. After sterilizing the area to be injected, the injector is set against the skin. Touching a small trigger forces the needle through the skin and then the patient pushes the plunger down, injecting the insulin. This device is not necessary for most people, who become very adept at self-injection.

"Jet injectors" are also available; these use no needles but force insulin through the skin with air under great pressure. A disadvantage is cost. Some jet injectors lack flexibility in the ability to vary doses and to use mixtures of insulin types. The injection is not totally without sensation. These devices are being improved technically and some patients find them satisfactory; however, they have not always delivered a consistent dose in the past.

> EVERY DIABETIC SHOULD BE PREPARED FOR EMERGENCIES, whether natural disasters, civil disturbances, or any other reasons. Always store some insulin and other necessary medicines. ROTATE SUPPLIES, USING OLDEST FIRST.

Injection Sites. The most common site for insulin injection is the thigh. Most people have enough flesh in this area and it is easy to reach. However, it is not desirable to continue injecting into the same site constantly, because the skin can become thickened and scarring can delay absorption. Also, lumps of fat may form underneath the skin, (a condition called "insulin hypertrophy").

Injection sites should be changed daily and rotated. If one places the injections in a straight line a little further down the thigh each day and then starts a second and third column, then moves to the other thigh, it will be several weeks before the injection returns to the first site. As seen in Figure 19, other possible injection sites are the upper arms and across the front of the abdomen as well as toward the sides. The abdomen is a good choice because it is easy to reach, is a vast area, and many patients have extra fat tissue there. Abdominal tissue is easy to grasp and if hollows caused by atrophy should occur, they are ordinarily not exposed to public view. The upper buttocks may be hard to reach but other members of the family could give injections there. Another way of reaching the buttocks is to lean back against a table edge or dresser so that the tissue is compressed firmly and is available as well. One should avoid injecting close to or below the knee or into the very outside of the thigh where the heaviest tissue is found.

The important thing is that injection sites should be rotated so that any area, an inch in diameter, is not used more often than once monthly if possible.

use of insulin to regulate diabetes

The principles of good regulation of diabetes are the same whatever the type of treatment. Insulin will always be effective if the proper dose is used. The ideal of treatment is to have

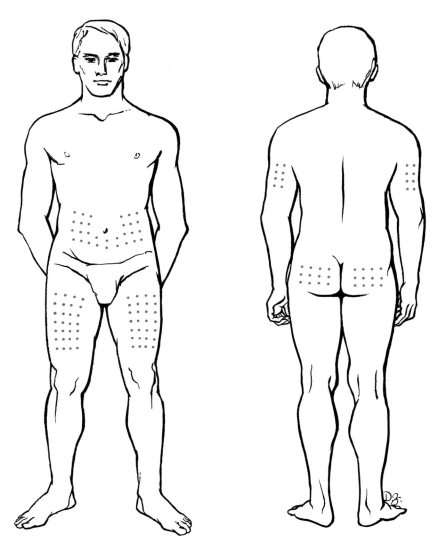

FIG. 19. Possible sites for insulin injection. Rotating injection sites helps to prevent the formation of atrophy, scarring, or hypertrophy. By using all the available sites, it may be possible to inject the same area no more than once a month.

enough insulin available to utilize or store food during the day, yet not so much insulin that increased activity causes insulin reactions. This degree of control is not always easy to achieve. Although the goal of treatment is to have a blood sugar level as normal as possible, this may not be easy, and sometimes it is impossible to achieve without multiple doses of regular insulin daily. Many patients tend to take too little insulin because they have an unsubstantiated suspicion that increasing the dose means that the diabetes is worse. Many fear reactions. Diabetes in some patients is so unstable that a change of only a few units of insulin one way or the other may make a vast difference in the degree of control. There is no way to equate insulin dosage to blood or urine sugar levels except by individual experience with each person. Each dose is determined by the patient's need and is important to that person, whether the requirement is 10 or 100 units daily.

Split Doses of Insulin.   Regular insulin is not commonly used as the only insulin because of its short action span; used singly, three or more injections would be required daily. However, multiple and well-chosen doses of regular insulin daily often provide the best control of diabetes, but not many patients would accept the inconvenience.

Because protamine zinc and Ultralente insulins are effective for too long a time (24 to 36 hours or more), the intermediate insulins, NPH and Lente, are used most commonly today. Although many patients, chiefly those who make substantial amounts of insulin in their own pancreases, require only one injection daily, other patients may find that NPH or Lente insulin is not effective for the full 24 hours. When this occurs, the morning blood and urine tests may show too much sugar despite satisfactory tests the rest of the day. It may then be necessary to use a *split dose* by taking roughly about three-quarters of the intermediate insulin before breakfast and a smaller dose, usually not larger than 25% of the total dose, before supper or at bedtime. If the diabetes is well-controlled in the morning, it will not require as much insulin during the day. Many physicians prefer split doses for the so-called brittle diabetics of all ages. (See Appendix 8 and Chapter 7, Timing of Urine Tests, p. 138.)

Adding Regular Insulin.   Other patients who use intermediate insulin find that the urine tests during the early part of the day, starting after breakfast and going till noon, show more sugar than desirable. They often are better regulated late in the day. This occurs because the intermediate insulin often has a slow starting action that permits the blood sugar level to rise before the insulin effect takes over. This problem is solved in many persons, particularly younger ones, by adding some rapidly-acting regular insulin to the morning intermediate dose, usually in a mixture of both insulins. This allows the fast-acting insulin to keep the blood sugar down until the intermediate insulin takes over later. These insulins can be placed in one syringe, drawing the regular insulin in first, and given in one injection.

In general, perfect control is not easily attainable in a patient who requires insulin. One common example of this is the difficulty of attaining normal blood glucose levels and avoiding sugar in the urine for several hours after breakfast. Too often the insulin effect does not appear soon enough after injection.

When combining the rapidly-acting regular insulin and an intermediate-acting insulin (NPH or Lente) in the same syringe, do not attempt to mix the insulin preparations in the bottle. As mentioned earlier, it is necessary to inject air into an insulin bottle (same amount as the insulin to be withdrawn) before one can withdraw the insulin. This breaks the vacuum that exists inside the insulin bottle. The same procedure must be done when drawing two types of insulin into one syringe, except that the rapidly-acting insulin is always drawn into the syringe first (*Fig. 20*).

1. Inject an amount of air equal to the dose of intermediate insulin into the NPH or Lente insulin bottle. Withdraw the *empty* syringe at this time without removing any insulin.

2. Ignore the previous bottle for the moment, inject an amount of air equal to the desired dose of regular insulin into that insulin bottle and remove the proper amount of regular insulin, getting out the bubbles as usual.

3. Return to the intermediate insulin bottle but do not inject any air this time. Simply insert the needle and withdraw the correct amount of NPH or Lente insulin.

4. This final amount in the syringe is the sum of the regular (crystalline) insulin plus the intermediate insulin for the total measured dose.

Patients become very adept at this procedure and have very little trouble with the technique.

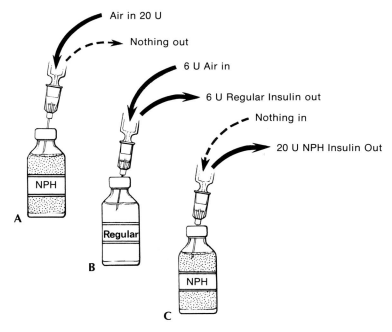

Air in 20 U

Nothing out

6 U Air in

6 U Regular Insulin out

Nothing in

20 U NPH Insulin Out

NPH

A

Regular

B

NPH

C

FIG. 20. Technique for mixing short- and long-acting insulins. In this example, 6 units of regular insulin and 20 units of NPH insulin are required.

factors affecting insulin effectiveness

It has been said that the "best laid plans of mice and men" often go awry. This is also true of insulin use. Many factors influence insulin effectiveness, including the following:

DIET.   Food intake is probably the most important factor affecting the insulin requirement. The amount of insulin needed may be halved or doubled by manipulation of diet. The insulin dose has little meaning unless a diet is also followed. This is a fact of life. Many patients, admitted to the hospital apparently requiring large amounts of insulin, need upon discharge doses that are only 25 or 50% of the amount previously required. Their first response is that the hospital insulin must be "different." The real reason is the food intake. For many people, the difference between requiring insulin or not simply depends on what, how much and when they eat.

EXERCISE.   Physical activity and exercise have a striking effect on insulin need. A remarkable difference occurs in a diabetic child's urine tests on a rainy, television-watching day as compared to an active, sunny day. At summer camps for children with diabetes, the urine test results, often negative for sugar on active days, are frequently + + + or + + + + on rainy days. This is one reason why school children sometimes need more insulin for school days compared to holidays and weekends, when they engage in heavy physical activity.

INFECTION OR ILLNESS.   The stresses caused by illness or infection have an important effect on the insulin dose. This includes fever, infection, surgery, or even common viral illnesses. These antagonize the insulin effect. More accurately, more body glucose and perhaps more glucagon are released, raising the requirement for insulin. (The use of insulin in these circumstances is discussed later under sick-day rules.) *Never* omit insulin in the face of illness or infection, because at such times more rather than less insulin often may be required.

INJECTION SITE.   The injection site greatly influences how rapidly or slowly insulin is absorbed and used. Injecting into scar tissue, hypertrophied fat or other areas with poor circulation slows the uptake of insulin. People who inject into more vascular areas will sometimes have reactions with the usual dose of insulin because the insulin may be more quickly absorbed in these areas.

OTHER MEDICATIONS.   Certain drugs and medications that are ordinarily proper and useful may unfavorably affect the blood sugar-lowering ability of insulin. For example, the effect of cortisone is well known. The use of these drugs may necessitate larger doses of insulin and often makes the regulation of diabetes more difficult. However, if such drugs are required, they should be used and the insulin increased as needed. Local injections of cortisone, as for bursitis of a shoulder, do not appear to affect diabetes significantly, nor does the application of cortisone as an ointment to the skin or as eye drops. Birth control pills and certain diuretic agents for the removal of body fluids also may increase the insulin requirement. A list of medicines that may affect the level of blood glucose is shown in Table 8.

TABLE 8. Commonly Used Medications That May Affect the Blood Glucose Level

Medications that tend to elevate the blood sugar level (decrease the insulin effect):

Epinephrine (Adrenalin)
Corticosteroids
Oral contraceptives
Anti-inflammatory agents such
   as Butazolidin
Thyroid replacement compounds
Cough syrups containing sugar

Diuretics such as:
   Diamox
   Dyrenium
   Edecrin
   Hygroton
   Lasix
   Other compounds with thiazides

Medications that tend to lower the blood sugar level (increase the insulin effect):

Alcohol, when taken internally
Certain antibiotics, such as Terramycin
Anticoagulants (dicumarol)
Monoamine oxidase inhibitors, which are used as antihypertensive agents (Eutonyl)
Propanolol, used in some cardiovascular conditions (Inderal)
Sulfonylureas
Salicylates, used as anti-inflammatory agents or for pain (aspirin)

* Although some of these compounds may affect blood sugar levels, your physician may have sound medical reasons for prescribing them. In some cases, the effect on the blood sugar level may be minimal or some medical effect is needed. Do not discontinue any medications without consulting your physician.

EMOTIONAL STRESS.   Emotional stress may increase the insulin requirement but its influence is often overrated. On a short-term basis, emergency situations may influence the release of epinephrine or cortisone by the body (both raise blood sugar). More importantly, under long-continued stress, people change their habits, including their eating patterns.

PHYSIOLOGIC STATES.   Certain physiologic states influence insulin doses. Noteworthy are menstrual periods, which sometimes require adjustments in the insulin dose or diet. Pregnancy increases the need for insulin until childbirth, when the requirement suddenly drops. Pathologic influences include overactivity of certain glands and other medical conditions that increase insulin need.

ANTIBODY FORMATION. Sometimes resistance to insulin caused by antibody formation makes insulin less effective. Although nearly all diabetics have some insensitivity to injected insulin, this resistance can become marked in certain patients.

Immune antibodies (which are described in Chapter 1), develop in the blood serum and bind the insulin, decreasing its effectiveness. This may occur for many reasons. Sometimes patients discontinue their insulin injections for a time, and then become allergic to the same protein (insulin) that was acceptable to them previously. The insulin preparations used today are products of other species of animals. All of them cause some antibody production in humans. For some reason, insulin made from beef causes slightly more antibody formation than that made from pork. Overweight also causes some insensitivity to insulin. When a tremendous insensitivity to insulin occurs, the condition is called insulin resistance. Most often this situation is not serious; it is often self-limited and is treatable.

adjusting the insulin dose

For Exercise. Those who undertake activities that are unusual for them may need to increase the diet or decrease the insulin dose. Unless the patient is very knowledgeable, both diet and insulin should not be changed at the same time. A good way to adjust for extraordinarily active work or activity (such as swimming or skiing) is to increase the food intake, utilizing more generous snacks. Some people who routinely sit at a desk during the week and become athletes on weekends may require two diets. This is also true of school children who need more food on play days. Sometimes the insulin dose may be reduced on activity days. In this situation, consult the patient's own physician, because he knows the patient well.

For Banquets and Parties. The insulin dose may have to be adjusted for banquets and parties, which often involve greater caloric intake than usual. The business dinner or banquet is now a part of our culture. The astute diabetic, realizing the need to attend a function in the evening, will have some portion of his supper at the usual time, or a bit earlier, and then have the rest of his food intake at the party. This may require injecting a larger dose of insulin or even an extra dose of regular insulin just before or after the party. Some experienced diabetics have been known to slip away from the festivities long enough to supplement their insulin; however, this is not an ideal approach for most persons.

For Long Auto Trips. The long automobile trip seems to be a normal part of American life. Although these prolonged periods of less activity increase the need for insulin, insulin reactions are a greater danger than some increased sugar in the urine. A driver who requires insulin must take small and frequent snacks to avoid the danger of an accident induced by a low blood sugar reaction.

Sick Days. Major, or even minor, illnesses probably cause the greatest problems and uncertainties for the diabetic. The most serious mistake made by diabetics during illness is decreasing or omitting their insulin dose because they "cannot eat." During such a period, even the usual dose of insulin may not be sufficient. Just as inflation reduces the buying power of money, two, three or more units of insulin may be needed to accomplish what one unit accomplishes normally. With illness, the patient may require *more* rather than less insulin. This certainly is the case when the urine tests show large amounts of both sugar and acetone. During illness, if the urine test is positive for sugar, *always check it for acetone.*

It may be necessary to take regular insulin every few hours until the urine tests improve. The amount of extra insulin depends on the usual daily dose. A rough rule is to take one-quarter of the usual 24-hour dose at intervals of four hours if the tests are + + + or + + + + for sugar in the urine. These sick-day rules are found in Appendix 7.

the ideal insulin dose

What is the ideal dose of insulin? No single perfect dose fits all people with diabetes. Diabetes is an individual condition and no two people are alike in their activities, metabolism or response to insulin. It would be just as logical for every woman to wear a size 12 dress or every man to wear a size 42 suit. The ideal dose is that which keeps blood sugar levels as close to normal as possible while permitting the patient to function free of insulin reactions. Note the words "as possible." With the insulin preparations now in use, it is sometimes necessary to compromise perfection for practicality. Success requires patience and changing insulin doses as needed. Perhaps the average dose ranges between 30 to 40 units daily. The "average" means nothing, though, because some (rare) people require several hundred units daily, while others have relatively good control with 10 or 12 units. It is estimated that 10% of the diabetic population takes as little as 10 units or less. Some of these are youngsters who will require larger doses as they grow. How much or how little insulin is used is not important—the ideal dose equals "enough"! It is important to recognize that in children, the more insulin that can be tolerated without having hypoglycemic reactions, the more normal and rapid growth will be. Normal growth cannot occur without adequate insulin.

Because the adjustment of the insulin dose is probably the most difficult and troublesome part of regulation, approximate rules for increasing and decreasing doses are found in Appendix 8. Of course, these rules are subject to the opinion of a person's own physician.

5

Oral
Hypoglycemic Agents

5

The tablets and capsules used to treat diabetes are known as oral hypoglycemic agents because they lower the level of the blood sugar. Their development has been one of the most exciting events since the discovery of insulin. These agents are not insulin, although patients sometimes make the mistake of thinking that they are.

Shortly after 1920 German scientists found a type of blood-sugar-lowering drug, but it had disturbing complications and these tablets were soon forgotten in the excitement surrounding the development of insulin. Dr. Elliott P. Joslin, while studying the effects of this early compound, Synthalin, made the shrewd prediction that while the medication was neither very effective nor useful, research would lead to further development of better oral medications that would be useful for diabetic patients. This new era started about 1955.

Many substances in nature have some ability to lower blood sugar levels. The problem is that these substances are not consistent in their action and some are not really very effective, while others are dangerous and toxic. When patients hear that someone has taken some herb that helped the diabetes, it is almost certain that some pharmaceutical company has tested this substance long ago. Many thousands of plants and compounds have been tried, including berry leaves, some types of raw cabbage and shrubs. Certain fruits as well as yams also have been known to have this effect.

Although it has already been emphasized, the importance of diet must again be stressed. Unfortunately, diet or meal planning is frequently neglected when oral agents are prescribed for patients. If blood sugar levels can be maintained near normal levels with diet alone, this is to be preferred. In general, oral agents should not be used for treatment until an adequate trial with suitable diet has been found to be ineffective.

the tablets are not insulin

Two types of oral agents have been effective in lowering blood sugar levels. Although neither is insulin, both depend on the presence of some insulin in the patient's pancreas to be effective. The sulfonylurea compounds are effective because they stimulate the release of insulin (*Fig. 21*). The other type, known as a biguanide (phenformin) is effective in ways that are not entirely clear but may include decreased absorption of sugars from the intestinal tract, lessened release of glucose from the liver and other organs, and a number of other effects that seem to help the body cells to utilize glucose (*Fig. 22*). The net effect seems to be that what little insulin the person has available in the body is made more effective. However, the biguanide compound phenformin is no longer available for general use, by order of the Food and Drug Administration, because of a serious possible side-effect known as lactic acidosis. It is now under strict FDA regulation and available only to certain patients in specific circumstances. (This ban on the use of phenformin is discussed more fully on page 115.)

When the sulfonylureas are effective, this means that the beta cells of the pancreas are able to react to the stimulation. Presumably, proper amounts of endogenous insulin (from a person's own pancreas) should be as useful as and indeed less antagonistic than injected insulin from another species (exog-

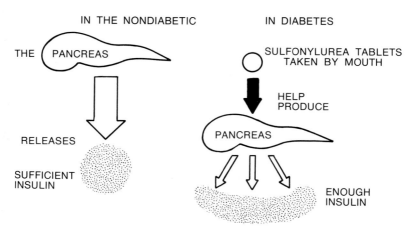

FIG. 21. Mechanism of action of the sulfonylurea oral compounds.

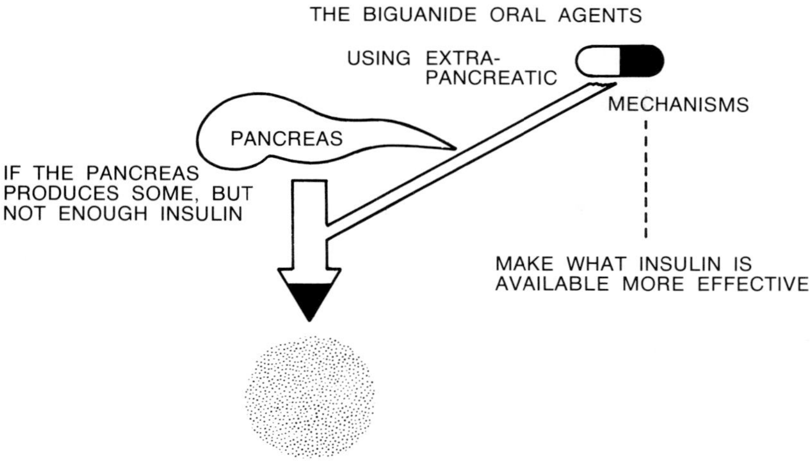

THE BIGUANIDE ORAL AGENTS

USING EXTRA-
PANCREATIC

MECHANISMS

PANCREAS

IF THE PANCREAS
PRODUCES SOME, BUT
NOT ENOUGH INSULIN

MAKE WHAT INSULIN IS
AVAILABLE MORE EFFECTIVE

FIG. 22. Mechanism of action of the biguanide oral compounds.

enous insulin). The paradox is that sulfonylurea tablets are most effective in normal (nondiabetic) persons, because in nondiabetics, the most insulin is available for release. The more severe the diabetes, the less insulin is produced. This reduces the effectiveness of these compounds.

Types of Available Oral Agents. The tablets available for treatment in the United States are shown in *Table 9* along with their main characteristics, usual dose, duration of action and other pertinent data. Although they are similar, the various sulfonylurea agents are not exactly identical. The general principle of action is similar, but their fate in the body and the effect of their metabolism determine their individual characteristics and effectiveness. These factors dictate the physician's preference in individual cases.

Tolbutamide (Orinase) is rapidly destroyed in the body and most of it is excreted in the urine in 24 hours. On the other hand, less than 1% of chlorpropamide (Diabinese) is metabolized and only 60% is excreted in 24 hours. This is why the latter compound has a much longer duration of action. Tolazamide (Tolinase) and acetohexamide (Dymelor), are intermediate in the duration of their action. Although Dymelor is rapidly used by the body, its use results in a byproduct (metab-

TABLE 9. Oral Hypoglycemic Medications in Use in the United States

	Generic Name	Trade Name	Manufacturer	Size	Usual Daily Dose
SULFONYLUREAS					
	Tolbutamide	Orinase	Upjohn	500 mg	500 to 2000 mg
	Tolazamide	Tolinase	Upjohn	100 mg 250 mg	100 to 1000 mg
	Chlorpropamide	Diabinese	Pfizer	100 mg 250 mg	100 to 500 mg
	Acetohexamide	Dymelor	Eli Lilly	250 mg 500 mg	250 to 1500 mg
BIGUANIDES*					
	Phenformin	Meltrol-25	USV Pharma-ceutical	25 mg	25 to 100 mg
		DBI-25	Geigy	25 mg	25 to 100 mg
	Phenformin, long-acting	Meltrol-50	USV Pharma-ceutical	50 mg	50 to 100 mg
		DBI-TD	Geigy	50 mg	50 to 100 mg

*No longer in general use by order of the Food and Drug Administration.

olite) that is two and one-half times more potent than the original tablet. Of course, by this time only minute traces are left, so usually the action subsides soon enough. Many other oral agents are in use in other parts of the world. One of these, glyburide (Glybenclamide), is widely used abroad. It has great blood-sugar-lowering ability with small doses. Five or ten milligrams of glyburide have the same effect as 500 to 1000 mg.

of tolbutamide (Orinase). Because diabetics often travel widely and trade names of medications vary internationally, the foreign trade names of the most common oral compounds appear in Appendix 9. However, it is best to carry a list of your medications that gives the generic (chemical) name while traveling, because pharmacists around the world understand these generic names.

who might use the oral compounds

The sulfonylurea compounds are effective only in persons who have a pancreas with beta cells capable of producing some insulin. Thus, most persons with long-standing diabetes, those who require large amounts of insulin, and very unstable diabetics, such as those of juvenile onset, are unable to use these compounds. These tablets are most effective in persons with recent-onset diabetes (usually less than ten years' duration), in the more stable group (those whose diabetes started after age forty), and in those who require less than 20 to 30 units of insulin daily. There are some exceptions to all of these general statements. Occasionally a longer-duration diabetic does respond to the oral agents. On the other hand, some patients who appear to meet all of the foregoing requirements find the tablets ineffective. There is never an "always" in medicine.

The *biguanides* have been generally useful for the same type of patients, although they do not increase the release of insulin. For this reason, some physicians had preferred them for overweight persons because, in theory, insulin is lipogenic (promotes fat deposition) and overinsulinization causes greater appetite and, indeed, more storage of fat. There is much disagreement about whether this is an advantage favoring the use of biguanide compounds.

Both types of oral agents may be ineffective during periods of stress, such as infection, injury or major surgical procedures. Under these circumstances many physicians change to the use of insulin, even if temporarily. The use of these oral compounds is not recommended during pregnancy because of possible harmful effects on the fetus. Moreover, at about the 36th week of pregnancy, the oral agents pass through the placenta to the fetus, thereby lowering the fetal blood sugar level.

combinations of oral agents

Since the sulfonylureas help the pancreas to release insulin and the biguanides potentiate the effects of insulin, a combination of the two types of drugs should be quite effective. Until the recent FDA action, this was the case for many diabetics.

Combining with Insulin. Generally speaking, combining insulin and oral agents has not proven effective. If oral agents can lower blood sugar levels, they do not need help. However, if they are ineffective, it is better to treat the patient with insulin alone. Rarely, patients have had their diabetes improved by using an oral agent along with insulin.

Mixing with Other Drugs. Some medicines used in the treatment of one disease can cause problems when mixed with other drugs or medicinal compounds (Table 10). This may occur with the oral blood-sugar lowering tablets. One of the more distressing problems occurs when some of the sulfonylurea compounds are mixed, not with medicine, but with alcohol. When these oral agents are taken along with alcoholic beverages, a strange phenomenon may take place. It is called the "Antabuse effect" (named after one of the common treat-

TABLE 10. Medications That Affect the Oral Hypoglycemic Agents		
	Increases Effect of Sulfonylurea	Increases Hypoglycemia
Alcohol*	X	X
Anticoagulants	X	
Butazolidin	X	
Chloromycetin	X	
Inderal		X
Ismelin		X
MAO inhibitor		X
Salicylates		X
Sulfonamides	X	

* Alcohol combines with sulfonylureas to cause an Antabuse effect (flushing of the face), in addition to causing hypoglycemia.
(Adapted from Medical Letter Inc., Vol. 19, No. 2, p. 8, 1977.)

ments for alcoholism). The blood vessels of the skin surface become sensitized and dilate, causing severe headache, nausea, and a redness or flushing of the face which, though harmless, is quite startling. The condition does not last long but can be alarming to the victim. Some medicines used by cardiac patients to delay blood coagulation, such as Coumadin, are affected by the sulfonylureas. Other medications, such as phenylbutazone (used for arthritis) and the common salicylates such as aspirin in large doses, have caused low-blood-sugar reactions when taken in combination with sulfonylurea compounds. Other drugs such as cortisone raise blood sugar levels and make the oral agents relatively ineffective. Some compounds that may affect the oral hypoglycemic agents are listed in Table 10. The safest course is to never take any new medication unless prescribed by the physician. *When in doubt about the use of any medication,* including those that can be obtained without prescription, *consult your physician.*

is diet still necessary

People sometimes wonder whether or not diet is still needed in this brave new world of oral agents. Diet is even more necessary. Insulin is more flexible than even the best of the oral agents, because the insulin dose can always be increased on demand. Oral agents have a fixed maximal effective dose. Doubling or tripling the dose beyond that point will not increase their effectiveness; it would be similar to adding more water to a full bathtub. Failure to adhere to diet almost certainly dooms the use of oral agents to failure.

DIET IS MORE IMPORTANT THAN EVER! Persons who take oral hypoglycemic agents often develop a false sense of security and neglect the diet. Since the oral compounds are not as effective as insulin itself, diet is even more important and may spell the difference between success and failure in this method of treatment for diabetes.

undesirable effects

Low Blood Sugar Reactions.   Anything that lowers blood sugar levels far enough can cause symptoms of hypoglycemic reactions. If sulfonylurea compounds release more insulin than required or if there is not enough body glucose available to meet the need, annoying "insulin-like" reactions are possible. Unusual exercise can also bring on this condition. Some of the longer-duration oral agents can cause severe reactions, although usually low-blood-sugar reactions with the tablets are not as severe as with insulin. For one thing, insulin is absorbed much more rapidly, and in many persons the amount of insulin released in response to oral agents is not great. However, meal plans and snack routines should be followed. Prevention and treatment are the same whatever the cause. By themselves, the biguanides did not cause reactions because they released no insulin.

Side Effects.   This is a term applied to symptoms that may result from taking any medication. Although certainly not desirable, they generally cause no real harm or permanent damage. Even generally "safe" drugs like aspirin can sometimes cause an upset stomach. Medicines containing codeine often affect people the same way. These effects usually stop when the dose is lowered or the medication discontinued.

The sulfonylurea compounds may cause side effects, but these are infrequent. Among these are gastrointestinal upsets, appetite loss, skin rash, itching and other undesirable symptoms that are relatively rare.

Side effects were more common with the biguanides. The most common problems were nausea and vomiting as a result of larger doses. Also frequently encountered were gas, a feeling of fullness, and diarrhea. Appetite loss (a strange phenomenon for most diabetics!) also was a common finding. These symptoms usually cleared up promptly when the medication was discontinued or the dose lowered.

Toxicity.   Toxicity is a much more serious effect; it may be lasting and possibly damaging. Many times good, accepted medications are occasionally "toxic" for certain individuals. For example, Chloromycetin, an antibiotic that can be lifesaving when used against typhoid fever and certain severe urinary tract infections, occasionally causes severe anemia. The physician, the pharmaceutical industry, and protective government agencies are eternally vigilant against toxicity. Considering the use of these oral medications by millions of diabetic patients around the world for more than 20 years, they have been extraordinarily free of toxicity. The sulfonylureas have been remarkable in this respect because evidence of acute toxicity has occurred only on rare occasions. In the presently used doses, changes in liver function have been rare.

The biguanides, although having a higher incidence of side effects than sulfonylureas, have been relatively freer of toxic effects. However, cases of lactic acidosis (an excessive accumulation of lactic acid) have occurred among patients who were treated with phenformin. Lactic acid is found normally in the body and excessive amounts are usually removed by the kidneys, liver, and other organs. Frequently, lactic acidosis causes death, and although the number of reported cases were few (about 300 to date) in comparison with the great number of diabetic persons who used phenformin daily (about 385,000), the Food and Drug Administration felt that the potential risks were not worth taking and ordered phenformin to be taken off the market as an "imminent hazard." However, phenformin is still available to some patients who cannot give themselves insulin or whose jobs are such that the risk of "insulin shock" would be a greater hazard than the possible hazard of phenformin. By FDA regulation, phenformin may be dispensed only by physicians who obtain IND (Investigative New Drug) certification and only in carefully prescribed circumstances.

the university group diabetes
program (UGDP) report

Physicians and their patients with diabetes have been disturbed during the past several years by a series of reports that suggest that oral hypoglycemic agents may be useless and possibly damaging. For 15 years there were no suggestions of complications caused by these widely used medications. In the summer of 1970, the University Group Diabetes Program (UGDP) investigators, who had observed the use of two of these oral agents (tolbutamide and phenformin) on selected patients from the large clinics of 12 university-affiliated hospitals, issued a report regarding tolbutamide and later one on phenformin. This report, unfortunately and inexcusably, was published widely in newspapers and magazines before publication in medical journals for evaluation of results by responsible physicians. The study involved a total of about 800 patients assigned to four treatment groups of 200 each. One group was treated with Orinase (tolbutamide), the only sulfonylurea used, with a fixed dose of 1.5 grams daily. Other groups received placebo (an inert, actionless pill), a fixed dose of insulin, or insulin as necessary. A group of somewhat similar size, added later, received phenformin. The patients chosen were those with recent onset of diabetes who might not have required specific treatment. The published reports indicated a much higher number of deaths from cardiovascular disease in those treated with tolbutamide.

An immediate furor arose at the time of the reports, and the controversy still rages on. Many physicians have disagreed with the UGDP findings, or with the interpretation of those findings. One report even suggested that the use of sulfonylureas had improved survival chances in patients who already had cardiac disease. It is true that the UGDP, with substantial federal funds available and with good scientific organization, was a *prospective* (planned in advance) study, while the others were *retrospective* (facts reported after they happened). Generally the prospective type of scientific study, if well-executed, is superior. At this point, the Food and Drug Administration (FDA), which rightfully has the job of protecting consumers, entered the controversy. This government agency (a) warned the physicians of the country of the results of this study; (b) tended to disregard the results of any studies that disagreed with the UGDP findings; (c) issued warnings about how the drugs should be used; (d) did not propose to remove them from use; and (e) after negotiations resulting from the controversy, for the time being left the use of these agents to the physicians' judgment, which is perhaps as it should be. The individual doctor is responsible for the treatment of his patients, and he should be alert to all facts, including those of the UGDP. Strong opposition arose from a group of diabetes specialists (Committee on the Care of the Diabetic) who disagreed, not necessarily with the findings of the UGDP, but with their interpretation. They also disagreed, not with the important responsibility of the FDA, but with that agency's acceptance of only one side of the argument. The report, although endorsed by the prestigious Biometric Society, has also been attacked on statistical grounds.

To date the UGDP implications have not been accepted by most responsible authorities throughout the world. The situation is unfortunate because of confusion among doctors and their patients. There is no question about the honesty or intent of the UGDP project, one of the best prospective studies to date. Their report shows that many persons receive diabetes medication needlessly; that properly used diet may be as effective as tablets; that inadequate treatment of any kind is no better than no treatment; that in later life, suboptimal treatment, as used in the study, does not protect against heart disease; and that among persons who live long enough, statistically many die from heart disease.

During the intervening years, some other studies have appeared to offer some corroborative information. Meanwhile, other studies from England and Sweden have disagreed completely with the original findings, and studies at the Joslin Clinic which, although retrospective, included thousands of patients observed for longer than 15 years, do not substantiate the UGDP impressions of great hazard to the heart and blood vessel system. The issue is further confused by the lack of definitive labelling regulations by the Food and Drug Administration. Hearings continue and the issue remains controversial. Suits in court were deemed necessary to protect the right of the physician to treat his patient as he considers best, but courts of law are not the ideal place for the settlement of scientific arguments; neither are the columns of newspapers. The *good* that might come from the discussion is the possible eventual gain from further research into better treatment. The *bad* is that many patients, and indeed their physicians, have been confused unnecessarily by the weighing of scientific evidence by nonmedical agencies.

In summary, it is safe to state that the situation regarding the ultimate use or usefulness of the oral hypoglycemic agents is still fluid. Phenformin has been banned from general use. Whether or not the views of the UGDP are eventually vindicated regarding sulfonylureas, a positive result has been the re-examination by many physicians of their beliefs concerning the use of any treatment. Too often the oral agents have been misused as a substitute for diet or prescribed in insufficient doses. Even the best oral agent has limitations, and once started, it is difficult to wean a patient from the easier approach to treatment. Although this oral aid to treatment of some types of diabetes appears to be useful, therapy must be adjusted to the needs of the individual patient and the optimal treatment should be used, whether or not it is the easiest to use or the most pleasant for the patient.

do the tablets become ineffective

Sometimes they do. This is called "secondary failure," assuming that the tablets were really effective in the first place. This success may be temporary; failure may be due to such factors as infection, surgery or severe injury. Many patients can resume treatment with the tablets satisfactorily when these conditions have been treated adequately. However, often it is found after varying periods of oral agent treatment that blood sugar levels become elevated and the physician has to increase the tablet dose. When this also fails, it may be due to "patient failure" as well as "pill failure." Patients may become careless with their diet. They may neglect to test for urine sugar and not realize that the dose is inadequate. Other patients deceive themselves by testing only the morning fasting urine, generally the best test of the day. They then assume that they are well regulated. If the oral agents really are inadequate for the job, insulin is needed. This may be temporary or permanent. Some wonder whether continued use of the tablets causes the pancreas to cease responding to stimulation, with results that resemble "whipping a tired horse." There is no evidence to indicate that such is the case. More than likely, the patient becomes tolerant to the drug, or in the natural history of diabetes, the condition simply worsens or requires more energetic treatment with the passing of time.

the good and the bad of oral medications

Barring any new information or more conclusive evidence of potential harm, the oral agents have some obvious advantages for patients in whom they are effective. Many patients find it

TABLE 11. Criteria for Measuring "Control" When Using Oral
Hypoglycemic Compounds (Blood Glucose in mg/100 ml)

Relation to Food	Good	Fair	Poor
Fasting	110	130	
1 hr p.c.	150	180	All other values
2 hr p.c.	130	150	
3 hr p.c.	110	130	

For classification of control as used by the Joslin Clinic, 70% or more of the blood glucose values
must conform with the listed standards.
The blood glucose values are determined with whole blood tested in the AutoAnalyzer.

difficult to take insulin. Anything that enables a large number
of people to be treated more simply is a great public health
boon, and in this respect the tablets have been a success.
Moreover, the development of these agents has stimulated
investigation leading to improved knowledge of diabetes.

There are also some disadvantages. The treatment is more
expensive than insulin treatment. The pills tend to make poor
control of diabetes easier because patients who start with oral
agents often resist treatment with insulin, postponing this
treatment to their own detriment. Some patients with severely
uncontrolled diabetes early in their course may have a better
chance for success with the oral agents if first treated with
insulin. At best, oral agents lack the flexibility of insulin.
Remember that each person is an individual whose diabetes
requires treatment designed specifically for him or her. The
welfare of the patient must come first, and the goal must
be the best control of the disease and greatest safety of the
patient.

What is "good control"? There should be no variance from
the goal that "normal" is best (*Table 11*). The best means of
achieving the goal for individual patients may vary, but the
objective, never!

the future of the oral agents

Medicine is a dynamic field of endeavor. Many medications
generate early enthusiasm that later becomes tempered with
reality. The really useful forms of treatment persist while

others fade into obscurity, to be replaced by something newer and better. The ideal oral agent for the treatment of diabetes (diet aside) has not yet been found; hopefully, newer more effective compounds will be found. The oral treatment of the future may not be the same as those available today. These are far from ideal. They are not effective at all in those who need them the most. While today's oral medications seek their place of true value in the court of scientific evaluation, they have given hope to many and proven not really effective enough for many more. Perhaps they are a phase in treatment, and at most, no more than another tool to be used properly and precisely. The ultimate oral agent would be a usable, low cost, easily available synthetic insulin that could be absorbed from the gastrointestinal tract. This goal does not appear to be within easy reach. Other oral agents are being constantly tested. The most widely used preparation outside of the United States is glyburide (Glybenclamide). If a compound other than those now available will be sanctioned, this is mostly likely to be the one. The future use of the present oral compounds depends on the outcome of the present controversy.

Meanwhile, some place in some laboratory, someone is working on other and newer means of treating diabetes by lowering the blood glucose level. Who knows what the future holds?

6

Other Factors
in Treatment

exercise

Exercise, whether at work or play, is as much a part of the treatment of diabetes as other forms of therapy. It is hard to overestimate its importance. For one thing, exercise helps to lower the blood glucose level. Some patients require much more insulin on days that they are sedentary than on days when they are very active. Adults have this problem because they may sit in an office during the week and then on Sunday play 36 holes of golf, ski or take part in other vigorous activities. This is even more obvious with children; on days when they are not in school, it may be necessary to increase their diet. There is also some evidence to suggest that the release of unidentified hormones may increase the metabolism of glucose during exercise. Studies at the Karolinska Institute in Stockholm show that, during exercise, there is much greater glucose release from the liver and uptake by muscles. This uptake of glucose by the leg muscles, for example, was higher than usual even if not enough insulin was available. This may explain why diabetics can have a lowered insulin requirement for several hours after the exercise stops. Another benefit of exercise is the increased uptake of free fatty acids.

Exercise, of course, must be suited to the individual's needs. For example, an hour of downhill skiing can use 500 calories, which would be a large amount for a person eating 1800 calories daily. All exercise need not occur in an organized method. Certainly, the mother of a large family, who is involved with care of her children and many household chores and who does a lot of walking, may get more exercise than someone involved with sport. Golf, for example, can be wonderful recreation and exercise, but an analysis of some golf foursomes, published in the *Smithsonian Magazine*, stated that the group spent 36.6% of their time walking and 8.5% of their time swinging (both good activities). However, they also spent 20.4% of the time standing motionless on the putting greens and 34.5% of the period simply waiting around. And they didn't even use a motorized golf cart.

Although exercise is important, the amount and type depends on physical health, the condition of the heart and other factors that must be considered in the decision about the proper amount of exercise. This must be determined by the patient's physician. Modern civilization has cut down physical activity for almost everyone; the overuse of automobiles, snowmobiles, power boats and other mechanized "sports" equipment, although not bad in themselves, permits a much lower expenditure of calories. Golf carts should be used only by people whose physical condition prohibits more active exercise.

Exercise doesn't have to be violent, but it should be consistent. How much exercise does a symphony conductor get? A study by a music-loving physician, Dr. L. Gordon of New York, showed that symphony conductors lead extraordinarily long lives and remain active, usually conducting, right up to the time of their deaths. This, of course, includes long hours of rehearsal. Walter Damrosch lived until 88; Toscanini, 89; Koussevitzky, 76; Pierre Monteux, 89; Beecham, 81; Casals, 94; Klemperer, 87. A number of prominent conductors still active are in their 70's and 80's. Possibly the exercise helps them to outlive the musician who sits in the orchestra. A British expert on aging states that ballerinas, cyclists and weight lifters also outlive those in sedentary pursuits.

Aside from the nonspecific "good health" reasons why exercise may prolong life, those who are vigorously active throughout life seem to have a much lower incidence of myocardial infarction. The very least the proper amount of exercise will do for you is to keep your body in tone, and, if you are healthy, it will help your heart, blood pressure and nearly all bodily functions. For the diabetic this aspect is even more important, because while food, stress and infection may be factors that favor the development of hyperglycemia, exercise tips the metabolic scales in the other direction.

Of course, there are more scientific reasons for the benefits of activity. For one thing, stored glucose in the liver is released much more readily. Exercise also affects insulin delivery to the muscle and its subsequent uptake and action on the muscle.

Since "fat" forms most of the displeasing bulges in overweight people and since fat (which provides 9 calories per gram) is the largest source of energy, it is encouraging to know that during heavy exercise fat is mobilized from storage depots in the body.

Studies in pre-insulin days showed that, when diabetes is greatly uncontrolled, the blood sugar level may rise rather than fall with exercise, because increased amounts of glucose are released from storage in the liver. Other studies have

TABLE 12. Energy Requirements of Common Activities

Activity	Cost in Calories per Minute*	Activity	Cost in Calories per Minute
Self-Care Activities		Housework	
Rest, supine	1.0	Hand sewing	1.4
Sitting	1.2	Sweeping floor	1.7
Standing, relaxed	1.4	Polishing furniture	2.4
Eating	1.4	Scrubbing, standing	2.9
Conversation	1.4	Washing small clothes	3.0
Dressing, undressing	2.3	Scrubbing floors	3.6
Washing hands, face	2.5	Making beds	3.9
Walking, 2.5 mph	3.6	Ironing, standing	4.2
Showering	4.2	Mopping	4.2
Walking downstairs	5.2	Hanging wash	4.5
Recreational Activities		Work Activities	
Painting, sitting	2.0	Sewing at machine	2.9
Driving car	2.8	Bricklaying	4.0
Horseback riding, (slow)	3.0	Plastering	4.1
		Tractor ploughing	4.2
Playing volleyball	3.5	Carpentry	6.8
Bowling	4.4	Mowing lawn by hand	7.3
Cycling, 5.5 mph	4.5	Shoveling	8.0
Golfing	5.0	Tending furnace	10.2
Swimming, 20 yd/min.	5.0		
Dancing	5.5	Master's Two-Step Test	8.2
Gardening	5.6		
Playing tennis	7.1		
Trotting horse	8.0		
Skiing	9.9		
Playing squash	10.2		

*To obtain calories per hour, multiply calories per minute by 60.
(From Gordon, E. E.: Energy cost of activities in health and disease. Arch. Intern. Med., 101:702, 1958. Copyright 1958, American Medical Association.)

shown that, while moderate exercise lowers the blood sugar level in both diabetics and nondiabetics, *true severe hypogly-cemia does not occur in nondiabetics.* That is, blood sugar levels can be lowered greatly in anyone who is exercising vigorously, as in marathon-running. However, the nondiabetic can utilize stored glucose and does not have the severely depressed levels of blood glucose that are found in diabetics who use too much insulin. The blood sugar level drops lower and remains low for a longer period in diabetics. One reason for this effect may be that the absorption of insulin from the depots where it is injected increases, owing to the exercise itself.

Table 12 shows how various types of exercise use calories. Remember that, while downhill skiing may use 500 calories an hour, cross-country skiing can help expend 1350 calories an hour. It is also much less expensive!

general hygiene

General body hygiene is such an important part of modern living that it is sometimes taken for granted. In the earliest editions of this book, written before insulin was used, Dr. Joslin devoted a whole chapter to hygiene for the diabetic. He included a number of topics such as exercise, proper rest, proper clothing, avoidance of overheated rooms (even before the "energy crisis"), general cleanliness, proper care of the teeth and the feet. These measures are still important. Long-term or inadequately treated diabetics are more prone to infection. The cleanliness of the skin may be the decisive factor in whether or not infection develops following a bruise.

Dental hygiene is particularly important. Dentists believe that badly controlled diabetes encourages disease of the gums, and they hesitate to perform dental surgery without proper regulation of the diabetes along with the administration of antibiotics. Diabetics, even more so than other persons, must take care of the teeth, which control the gateway to the gastro-intestinal tract.

Foot Care.   Foot care is discussed in Chapter 9. Improper foot care is one of the leading causes of disability in older persons with diabetes.

education of diabetics

Education is a goal to which nearly everyone aspires. It is almost impossible for those with diabetes to cope with modern life without comprehensive knowledge of their condition. Education is not an addition to treatment—it is treatment! No one can be adequately treated for diabetes without being taught the fundamentals of diet, technique of insulin injection, treatment of low blood sugar levels, foot care and a half-dozen other subjects that help a diabetic survive. Those long-term diabetics who have survived best are those who knew the most. No matter how often a diabetic sees his or her physician, whether it be four or more times yearly, the fact remains that the person with diabetes must live with that disease 60 minutes an hour, 24 hours a day, 365 days a year, and now frequently for 50 or more years! If a person requires two injections of insulin daily, the total number of injections amounts to about 750 a year, 7,500 in ten years, and almost 23,000 in 30 years. Not only his comfort but his very survival depends on knowledge. No hospital can be considered first-class without providing a teaching program for diabetics.

This section has dealt with certain forms of treatment which, though nonspecific, are nonetheless important. Perhaps these items count as only small percentages of the total treatment program, but these are very important percentages. These factors can make the difference between success and failure in living the best possible life with diabetes.

7

Testing

The best way to ensure success for the person with diabetes is frequent testing for sugar in the urine and periodic testing for the level of sugar in the blood. Testing is probably the best life insurance available for diabetics. Some people put a lot of stock in reading tea leaves for telling their fortune. Reading urine tests is more useful, at least for the diabetic.

An important question is how frequently a person with diabetes should have blood and urine tests performed. As far as blood sugar levels are concerned, this depends entirely on the advice of the physician who is responsible for the patient. Determining factors may include the ease with which the diabetes is regulated and the intelligence and cooperation of the patient. Early, while regulation of the diabetes is being determined by educated trial-and-error, blood sugar tests should be performed frequently. Later, blood sugar tests performed possibly every three months or so would be a desirable schedule, depending entirely on the person's individual pattern. Urine tests must be done much more frequently and many patients need to do them three or four times daily, before meals and at bedtime. They are simple to do accurately and provide a guide to the patient's course of therapy. However, these procedures should not merely be a ritual, but for the purpose of determining the degree of regulation of the diabetes.

testing blood for sugar

Because an objective of treatment is to keep the blood sugar as close to normal levels as possible, obviously blood sugar tests are the most important measurement of diabetes regulation. Other measures are blood levels of cholesterol and fat, body weight, and a sense of well-being. The urine sugar test is also important, but it lags behind the blood glucose by several hours. After a person eats or drinks, the blood sugar level increases and reaches its peak about one-half to one hour later. It may be two hours or more before the results of this meal are reflected in the urine sugar values. For example, if a person eats breakfast at 8 a.m., the blood sugar level reaches its peak usually at 9 a.m.; glucose, if any, will appear in the urine at 10 a.m. and later, at which time the blood sugar level is dropping.

This same sequence of events also happens to nondiabetics, except that because they have sufficient insulin, the blood sugar levels never go above normal. Using a true glucose value in *whole* blood, the normal fasting blood level is about 60 to 100 mg. per cent. One hour after eating (also known as postcibal or postprandial), the normal value may range from 100 to 140 mg. per cent (venous whole blood). Rarely does the blood sugar go above 150 mg. per cent in a nondiabetic, although a high value is usually not considered suggestive of diabetes until it reaches 160 mg. per cent. In two hours, the blood sugar level in normal individuals is no higher than 80 to 120 mg. per cent, and very rapidly thereafter it returns to the fasting level. Levels of plasma glucose (now used in many hospitals and clinics) are about 15% higher than whole blood readings.

All the levels mentioned previously are for blood taken from a vein. When capillary blood is taken from the finger pad or ear lobe, its sugar content approximates that of arterial blood, and after eating the blood glucose level usually runs between 20 and 30 mg. per cent higher than in venous blood. The arterial (or capillary) blood contains more glucose because it is on the way to the cells with nourishment, while the venous blood has less glucose because it is on the return trip. The values should be about the same in the fasting state.

An older method of blood sugar determination, used in some places, is called the Folin-Wu method. It yields values which on the average are about 20 mg. per cent higher than the true glucose values. The normal fasting value is between 80 and 120 mg. per cent (*Table 13*).

Nondiabetics have such tremendous insulin-producing capacity that only about 5% of the population ever have elevated blood glucose levels. Diabetics do not have enough available insulin, so that their levels of blood glucose are often considerably higher.

TABLE 13. Comparison of Diagnostic Standards for Blood Glucose
Tests, Using the Folin-Wu Method and the
"True Sugar" Method.

Relation to Food or Glucose Ingestion	Folin-Wu	"True Sugar"	
		Venous	Capillary
Fasting	130	110	110
Normal Fasting	80-120	60-100	60-100
1 hour	170	160	190
2 hours		120	150
3 hours		110	110

All values in mg. per cent. The "true sugar" levels are with whole blood; many institutions use plasma, which may be 10% to 15% higher.
These figures are for detection or diagnosis; more ideal levels for treatment are shown in Table 11.

One factor that determines how often a person should have blood sugar tests performed is the relationship between blood and urine sugar levels. In the very young, sugar tends to appear in the urine at much lower blood glucose levels. Sometimes urinary sugar appears even with normal blood sugar levels. In older persons, the ability to excrete excess glucose from the blood by way of the kidney diminishes. This means that some older people can have fairly high blood sugar levels without much glucose appearing in the urine. At the other end of the scale, if a child with diabetes consistently has sugar-free urine, there is a threat of hypoglycemic reactions because the blood glucose level may be low during "normal" urine sugar tests.

The term "renal or *kidney threshold*" confuses a lot of people needlessly. It simply refers to the way in which the kidney retrieves the glucose that is important for the nourishment of the person from filtered blood. If there is more glucose than the kidney can handle, it spills over into the urine and is voided. The level at which sugar generally spills over is between 160 to 170 mg. per cent. The kidney threshold is like a dam that holds back water until its capacity is exceeded. This critical point varies somewhat and is never completely constant. It may be necessary to obtain several blood sugar readings several times daily to determine the guidelines needed to help the doctor and the patient know which tests to use and how often. If a person has reasonably stable diabetes, a blood sugar test performed once every few months may be sufficient. Others may require a blood sugar test every few weeks or even every few days during unstable periods.

Nondiabetics rarely have any sugar in the urine, except in a nondiabetic condition known as renal glycosuria, in which sugar appears in the urine even at low levels of blood glucose.

Dextrostix. A reasonably simple method that can roughly estimate the "true glucose" content of blood is now available. This is called Dextrostix.* Chemically treated plastic strips give an approximate level of "true sugar" after 60 seconds with one drop of capillary blood from the ear lobe or fingertip. Certain precautions will ensure accuracy. Sterile technique with a small lancet is important. A color chart measures blood sugar levels from 40 to 250 mg. per cent. The color changes from intense shades of gray to blue, depending on the amount of sugar present in the drop of blood. However, many find it difficult to differentiate shades of blue or gray. Also, since the gradations are approximately 50 mg. apart, an error in technique or reading can make a considerable difference. Recently the company has introduced a "reflectance meter" that is designed to give more accurate readings when used with Dextrostix. It is a small, lightweight instrument powered with a rechargeable battery, and it is reasonably accurate if the person using it is meticulous. The device is relatively expensive for home use and is probably most useful in a clinic or physician's office, although occasionally highly motivated patients have found it useful. While most diabetics do not have to use Dextrostix as a method for measuring blood glucose levels precisely, this test may be useful for generally indicating whether the blood sugar level is very high or very low. This may be helpful with children, because their symptoms may be difficult to interpret and one may not be certain whether the blood sugar is low, normal or high.

testing urine for sugar

For most diabetics, the most practical way of judging the status of diabetes is by urine tests. The most common useful

* Manufactured by Ames Company, Elkhart, Indiana.

tests are those for urine sugar and acetone. Urine sugar testing is simple and inexpensive, and, when properly used, can give enough information to guide treatment. Unfortunately, urine testing is so easy to perform that patients often neglect it. The purpose of the test is to determine the amount of sugar present in the urine, as a guide to increasing or decreasing the insulin dose as needed. If sugar is present in significant amounts, then an acetone test should be done to determine how badly the diabetes may be out of control. In busy modern life, urine testing is easy to overlook. When diabetes is really stable, it may not be necessary to test as often. Certainly, all diabetics whose regulation is poor and most juveniles need to test frequently.

URINE TESTING IS VITAL.

Although it is often an unpopular procedure for many diabetics, it provides important information. The purpose is not to impress your physician with a sheet full of "zeros" for sugar, but to provide information to guide your treatment. Especially with youngsters, tests should not be described as "good" or "bad." It is not a moral issue, but rather shows how much glucose (fuel for the body) is being retained or lost.

However, the patient must remember certain points. Although a urine test may be "negative" for sugar, the test may not indicate how low the blood sugar level is. Sometimes experienced diabetics claim they are able to differentiate "degrees of normal" by the depth of color.

The first urine test performed in the morning, or after long periods of not urinating, is not always accurate as an estimate of the current blood sugar level, because the urine may have been stored in the bladder for a number of hours. The most accurate method of testing is to discard the first urine specimen, drink a glass or two of water, and a half-hour later get a second urine specimen to test. In other words, one should not test the first urine voided after the taking of food. This explains why it is possible for a person to be in hypoglycemic reaction (have a low blood sugar level) while the urine shows the presence of considerable amounts of sugar. The answer is simply that the urine specimen was formed by the kidneys when the blood sugar was high and it remained in the bladder for some time.

Therefore, two good reasons for urine testing are: (1) poor tests may indicate that more insulin is needed; (2) tests that are consistently free of sugar may, although not invariably, indicate the need for reduction in insulin dose to avoid possible reactions.

types of tests

There are many tests available, ranging from Benedict's test (formerly used almost exclusively) to more modern strip methods. They vary in accuracy, difficulty of performance, cost and interpretation. It is not so much which test is used as how it is used. The various available tests are shown in Appendix 10. The most common ones currently in use are Clinitest, five- and two-drop method (Ames), Tes-Tape (Lilly), Diastix (Ames), and Clinistix (Ames). Actually, Diastix is replacing Clinistix, which has less precise levels. For those with impaired vision, Mega-Stix (Ames) has larger areas of color for easier reading. Some diabetics still use the old-fashioned but dependable Benedict's test. The techniques for these tests are briefly outlined in Table 14. Each type of test has its champions. Reporting *colors* to the physician is not desirable, because blue may mean no sugar with one test and much sugar with another type of test. The patient must read the instructions carefully, and it is better to record the result as "per cent" rather than as "plus signs" or colors.

Table 15 compares several of the most common tests available. *Tes-Tape* is convenient for determining whether a urine specimen is sugar free or contains sugar. In comparison with Clinitest or Benedict's tests, Tes-Tape has two major limitations: its great sensitivity in low urine sugar concentrations, and abrupt jumps in readings from $\frac{1}{2}\%$ ($+++$) to 2% ($++++$). The tape must be used carefully because it can be inactivated by aging or high humidity, and a patient can be falsely reassured by an inactive tape test or dip stick. Chemstrip G (Boehringer) is a new strip test. The colors are easy to read, but large doses of vitamin C present in the urine may

TABLE 14. Tests for Sugar in the Urine

	Color	Per Cent Sugar	Record
I. CLINITEST* 5-drop method			
1. 5 drops urine ⎫	Blue	0	0
2. 10 drops water ⎬ combine	Green	$\frac{1}{4}\%$	Trace
3. 1 Clinitest tablet ⎭	Cloudy Green	$\frac{1}{2}\%$	1+
4. Wait 15 seconds after	Olive Green	$\frac{3}{4}\%$	2+
boiling stops	Yellow to Light Brown	1%	3+
5. Shake gently, compare	Orange	2%	4+
with color chart	Orange to	—more than	
	Greenish-Brown	2%**	
II. CLINITEST* 2-drop method			
(for greater than 2% sugar)	Blue	0	0
1. 2 drops urine ⎫	Green	$\frac{1}{4}\%$	Trace
2. 10 drops water ⎬ combine	Cloudy Green	$\frac{1}{2}\%$	1+
3. 1 Clinitest tablet ⎭	Olive Green	1%	2+
4. Wait 15 seconds after	Yellow Brown	2%	3+
boiling stops	Light Brown	3%	4+
5. Shake gently, compare	Orange	5%	5+
with color chart			
III. TES-TAPE			
1. Withdraw approxi-	Yellow	0	0
mately $1\frac{1}{2}$ inches of	Light Green	1/10%	1+
tape	Dark Green	$\frac{1}{4}\%$	2+
2. Dip end of tape in	Dark Green to Blue	$\frac{1}{2}\%$	3+
specimen of urine. Re-	Dark Blue	2% or	4+
move and wait exactly		more	
one minute.			
3. Then immediately			
compare the darkest			
area with color on dis-			
penser. Unchanged			
yellow color indicates			
urine is sugar free. If			
tape indicates $\frac{1}{2}\%$ or			
greater, wait one addi-			
tional minute and			
make final comparison.			
IV. DIASTIX			
1. Dip strip in urine for 2	Blue	0	0
seconds	Light Green	1/10%	Trace
2. Tap strip to remove	Dark Green	$\frac{1}{4}\%$	1+
excess	Olive Green	$\frac{1}{2}\%$	2+
3. Compare strip to color	Light Brown	1%	3+
chart in approximately	Dark Brown	2%	4+
30 seconds			

TABLE 14. Tests for Sugar in the Urine (Continued)

	Color	Per Cent Sugar	Record
V. BENEDICT'S TEST			
1. 4 drops of urine in test tube	Blue	0	0
	Pea-Green	1/10%	1 +
2. add ½ tsp (2.5 cc) of Benedict's solution†	Yellow-Green	½%	2 +
	Yellow or Brown	1%	3 +
3. shake tube; place in boiling water for 5 minutes	Red	2%	4 +
4. remove from water and examine			

Alternate method:
1. 8 drops of urine in test tube
2. add 1 tsp (5 cc) of Benedict's solution
3. using tube-holder, heat over an open flame. (Do not let the mixture heat too fast, because the urine will boil over.)
4. remove from heat and examine

	Color	Per Cent Sugar	Record
VI. CHEMSTRIP G			
1. Mix 1 part of urine and 3 parts water (such as 5 drops of urine and 15 drops of water).	Yellow	0	0
	Orange	1/10%	1 +
	Pink	½%	2 +
	Red-Brown	1%	3 +
	Brown	2%	4 +
2. Dip plastic stick into urine for 1 second.			
3. If color does not change after 1 minute, test is negative for sugar.			
4. If color does change after 1 minute, wait 4 minutes and then compare with color chart on bottle.			

NOTE: The use of plus signs to denote percentage of glucose contained in specimens is purely arbitrary. Moreover, the colors indicating test results differ according to the test. Therefore, patients should report test results in terms of percentages only.

* Clinitest reagent tablets will absorb moisture and spoil (turn dark blue) if the bottle is not closed tightly.

** Rapid Pass Through—see Clinitest color chart.

† Benedict's solution is a stable compound that does not decompose even after months. It can be obtained from your pharmacist.

TABLE 15. Comparison of Clinitest, Tes-Tape, and Diastix

Per Cent Urine Sugar	0	1/10	¼	½	¾	1%	2%
Clinitest	0	0	Trace	1+	2+	3+	4+
Tes-Tape	0	1+	2+	3+			4+
Diastix		Trace	1+	2+		3+	4+

Clinistix does not readily fit into this table because the presence of sugar is indicated only by light, medium and dark shades of purple.

cause errors in the test result. This testing device probably has no significant advantage over the other urine test materials.

Each of these urine tests has to be compared with its own color chart for accurate interpretation. The patient should make certain that he and his physician are talking about the same test method and means of recording. Other factors affecting the choice of test are the convenience of one test as compared with another and their comparative simplicity and relative costs (*Table 16*). More important, the patient must learn the technique thoroughly and understand the test used.

Although no test is perfect, the tablet, tape or strip tests are convenient and many prefer them. Some use the strip or tape test while traveling and either the tablet or Benedict's solution at home. Although many consider it cumbersome, the old-fashioned Benedict's test is still a standard, dependable urine test that is inexpensive.

Two-Drop or Five-Drop Tests? Many people are confused about the difference between the regular five-drop Clinitest and the two-drop Clinitest methods. With the regular five-drop Clinitest method, loss of sugar in the urine greater than 2% (4+) cannot be measured. In fact, if the urine sugar is higher than 2%, the reaction goes through the color ranges much too quickly.

The two-drop method is most often used for unstable or juvenile type of diabetes. It uses two drops of urine instead of five. This results in a different ratio of urine to water and a special chart allows recognition of much higher levels of sugar (over 2%) by matching the color against the color chart. The

TABLE 16. A Shopper's Guide to Urine Testing Materials

Test	Advantages	Disadvantages	Assessment
Clinitest (Ames)	Color changes easy to read. No false negatives.*	Some medications cause false positives.† Second least convenient for travel (requires bottle, test tube, dropper, urine receptacle).	Less convenient than tape and strip tests. Not most expensive. Easily readable colors. Some false positives. Never false negatives.
Tes-Tape (Lilly)	Most convenient, especially for travel. Slightly less expensive than other tests, except Benedict's solution.	Not accurate with high glucose levels. Under-reads 2% (4+) Some medications cause false negatives.	Probably lowest cost, except for Benedict's solution. Most convenient. Read 3+ as 4+. Some false negatives. No false positives.
Diastix (Ames)	Colors easy to read. Convenient for home and travel.	Most expensive. Some medications cause false negatives. Sometimes under-reads high glucose level.	Most expensive. Convenient. More accurate than Tes-Tape; less accurate than Clini-test. Some false negatives. No false positives.
Benedict's solution	Lowest cost by purchasing large containers of solution. Colors easy to read.	Cumbersome. Positive for sugars other than glucose.	Cheapest. Clumsy; almost impossible for travel. Some sugars other than glucose can cause false positives.
Chemstrip G	Colors easy to read. Stiff plastic stick holds together well.	Expensive. Large doses of Vitamin C give false results.	Newest device. Convenient, but no definite advantage over other tests.

*A false negative result misses glucose when present.
†A false positive result indicates glucose when not present.
(Adapted from Seltzer, H.S.: Urinary glucose tests. Diabetes Forecast, 30:27, 1977.)

five-drop method is satisfactory for most persons with diabetes, but those, such as juveniles, who are likely to run higher sugar levels can obtain more reliable results with the two-drop method.

Timing of Tests. The information given by tests depends on their timing (*Table 17*). (1) *Before breakfast.* This test tells whether the effects of intermediate (NPH or Lente) insulin administered the previous morning have continued through the night. If the tests are unsatisfactory, more insulin may be needed. If patients take supplemental insulin before supper or at bedtime, the early morning test indicates whether this dose is adequate. (2) *Before the noon meal.* This test indicates the diabetes state since breakfast. Some people lose extraordinary amounts of glucose in the urine before the intermediate insulin becomes effective. Some regular insulin may be needed before breakfast, or if the patient is already taking such, an increase in dose may be indicated. (3) *Tests before the evening meal* indicate whether the dose of NPH or Lente insulin taken

TABLE 17. Insulin Changes Based on Tests for Glucose in Blood and Urine.*

Before Breakfast	Before Lunch	Before Supper	Bedtime	Adjust Insulin
+	+	+	+	increase morning intermediate dose
0	+	0	0 ⎫	may need added
0	+	+	0 ⎭	morning crystalline
0	0	+	0 ⎫	increase morning
0	0	+	+ ⎭	intermediate dose
0	0	0	+	decrease supper carbo-hydrate or add some crystalline before supper
+	0	0	0 ⎫	may need some intermediate
+	+	0	0 ⎭	at supper or bedtime

0 = normal level of glucose in blood or urine specimen.
+ = significantly elevated level of glucose in blood or urine specimen.
*Change insulin dosage only with the advice and consent of your physician.
Changes in insulin dosage usually involve no more than 2 units at a time, and usually only when elevated test results appear consistently for several days. (See also Chapter 4, p. 96 and Appendix 8.)

before breakfast is adequate or not. (4) *Bedtime tests* determine whether the insulin taken in the morning is active long enough for the patient to utilize food eaten at supper. Table 17 summarizes this. (See also p. 96 and Appendix 8.)

Twenty-Four-Hour Urine Test. A very useful test for many diabetics is the 24-hour quantitative test. Some physicians suggest that this test be performed every two to four weeks. Ideally a person would lose no sugar in the urine in 24 hours; in any case, good regulation for adult-onset type of diabetes would mean no loss greater than 5% of the total carbohydrate intake for the day (e.g., with 200 grams of carbohydrate in the diet there should be no more than 10 grams lost). With children, a maximum loss would be 10% of the daily carbohydrate intake, or 20 grams with a diet of 200 grams of carbohydrate daily. The technique for this is described in *Table 18.*

TABLE 18. Testing for Sugar in a 24-Hour Specimen

1. Certain physicians suggest that this test be done every two weeks for children and once a month for adults.
2. Ideally, the result of this test should show no sugar and in no case should adults show more than 5% of the total carbohydrate allowance for the day (180 grams CHO, 9 grams sugar). Children should not lose more than 10% of their carbohydrate allowance.
3. *Procedure*
   a. Collect 24-hour specimen by discarding the first voided specimen and saving all specimens for 24 hours, including first voided the next morning. This must be measured for amount in ounces.
   b. Change the ounces to milliliters* by multiplying by 30 (1 ounce = 30 ml).
   c. Take a specimen of the total amount and test with Clinitest. Find the per cent of sugar in the specimen.
   d. Multiply the total milliliters by the per cent of sugar found from the Clinitest. This will give you the grams of sugar lost in a 24-hour period.
   e. Report this information to the doctor.

Example: 40 ounces
        40 ounces × 30 ml = 1200 in total milliliters*
                ×   .01 (1% sugar from Clinitest chart)
           12.00 grams of sugar lost in the
              24-hour period

*1 ml = 1 cc

testing urine for acetone

The urine test for acetone is not done as frequently as the test for glucose but it can be vital. Calories are provided for energy from the proper breakdown of carbohydrate in the presence of adequate insulin. If there is a shortage of insulin, fat is broken down into ketones, which include acetone and betahydroxy-butyric acid. Acetone may be found in the urine under certain conditions, such as fever or overactivity on a hot day without adequate carbohydrate intake. Significant amounts of ketones in the urine of a diabetic almost always indicate trouble. As the control of diabetes worsens, from whatever cause, increasing amounts of acetone appear. This trend can be reversed by adequate treatment. If unchecked, the acetone becomes more marked and may be a precursor to diabetic ketoacidosis or even diabetic coma. The finding of acetone in the urine must never be ignored! Several testing methods are described in Table 19. Although urine testing is one of the simplest procedures, some surveys have shown that less than 5% of patients knew how or why to test for ketones.

URINE ACETONE TESTS ARE IMPORTANT and should always be done when large amounts of sugar are present in the urine.

Don't panic about one poor test result! Repeat the test. Some patients become so upset by one poor test result that they overreact. The insulin dosage should not be changed on the basis of one poor test. Some physicians prefer several days of testing before changing insulin doses. *Ask your doctor!*

influences on blood and urine sugar levels

Blood sugar levels are influenced by many factors besides the dosage of insulin. As described earlier, many medications can increase blood sugar levels. These include thiazides, oral con-

TABLE 19. Urine Tests for Acetone

Test	Color	Acetone Present
Acetest Method		
1. Place white Acetest tablet on clean white paper or a paper towel.	No change Lavender	None Small amount
2. Put a drop or two of urine on the tablet.	Light purple	Moderate amount
3. Read color change at end of 30 seconds (no longer). Color chart supplied with each bottle of tablets.	Dark purple	Large amount
Ketostix Method		
1. Dip test end of strip in urine.	Same as above.	Same as above.
2. Compare with color chart 15 seconds after dipping.		
Keto-Diastix Method		
1. Dip test end of strip in urine.	Same as above.	Same as above.
2. For ketones, compare with color chart 15 seconds after dipping.		
3. For glucose, compare with color chart 30 seconds after dipping. (Some patients find this test confusing. Because ketone testing is not necessary with every urine test, this device is not necessary for routine testing.)		

It is not necessary to test the urine for ketones daily.
It is important, however, to test for ketones as well as sugar when:
1. urine tests are consistently 4+ or greater for two consecutive tests.
2. acute illness occurs, especially when fever is present.
3. episodes of nausea and vomiting are noted.
4. surgery, injury or other stress has occurred.
5. insulin dosage is being adjusted.
6. treatment with oral blood-sugar-lowering agents is being started.

traceptive agents, glucagon, thyroid extract, estrogen, cortisone and epinephrine. Caffeine in large amounts may have the same effect, as well as infection and pregnancy. Many of these factors do not change the blood sugar to a great extent. Certain compounds, such as aspirin in very large doses, some of the drugs used to prevent blood coagulation, sulfonamides, barbituates, alcohol, and antihistamines, as well as strenuous exercise and insufficient food, may lower blood sugar levels.

Urine tests can also be misleading through the influence of other substances. Lactose, which appears in the urine of lactating mothers, may cause a positive Clinitest reaction even in the absence of glucose. Aspirin in large doses may cause falsely negative strip tests, as can large doses of vitamin C. Certain antibiotics may give a false color to the Clinitest and a false positive result for other tests. Not all of these errors are significant, but such test results may be misleading unless the patient is aware of the possible effects.

Most errors are caused by poor testing technique. The commonest cause of miscalculating the amount of sugar in the urine is diluting with too much urine or water.

In summary, all of these tests are useful. None is perfect. When in doubt, consult your physician.

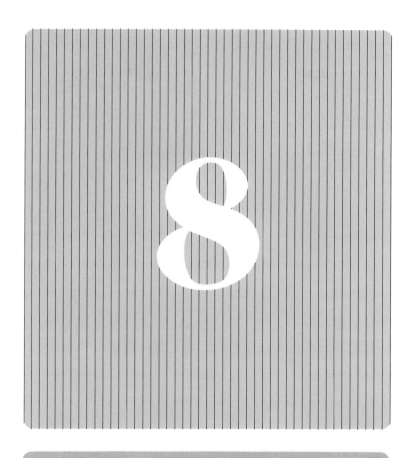

8

Acute Complications

8

Even under the best of circumstances, the course of diabetes, like "the course of true love," may not run smoothly. Its natural history has been discussed earlier. However, all cases of diabetes do not run this same course. Just as there is no "typical" person, there is no "typical diabetic." Diabetes is an individual condition that varies with each person. It is difficult to predict a specific course for any given patient. In adults, the onset can be very insidious. Many people have active and recognizable diabetes for years before it is actually noticed or diagnosed. This may be why, in an occasional case, complications are present at the time of initial diagnosis. On the other hand, occasionally older persons have an abrupt onset very much like that of the so-called juvenile diabetic. Juvenile diabetes is most often announced with a blare of symptomatic trumpets and is difficult to miss. For many children, the diabetes is discovered when they have developed ketoacidosis. However, increasingly it is believed that some young people may also have an adult type of diabetes, with gradually increasing blood sugar levels long before the symptoms develop and the condition becomes obvious.

More than with many medical conditions, the treatment of diabetes can influence its course. When the overweight diabetic with elevated blood sugar levels loses weight, often the diabetes seems to disappear. "Seems to disappear" is the proper statement, because the basic diabetic condition lurks beneath the surface and comes to the fore with dietary indiscretion, infection or regaining weight, or simply with the passage of time and slowly progressive inability of the beta cells to function well.

144

early or late complications

These terms are used loosely, especially since the "early" complications are those that can and do occur anytime during a diabetic lifetime.

Some diabetes complications are neither disabling nor permanent. The *early complications* are acute situations that can appear anytime, even early in the course of diabetes, and are usually remediable. The most important are (1) hypoglycemic (insulin) reactions and (2) diabetic ketoacidosis or coma. The *late complications,* or long-term complications, are discussed in Chapter 9. Much present research is directed toward this group of complications. These conditions are usually more serious than early complications.

hypoglycemia (insulin reaction)

Hypoglycemia simply means a low blood sugar level. Although there are several types or causes of hypoglycemia, the discussion presented here concerns one of the most common complications for diabetics—low blood sugar level resulting from overtreatment with insulin or oral hypoglycemic agent, from insufficient food intake, or from exercise that is exceptional for the individual. Few well-controlled diabetics who have used insulin for any length of time can say that they have never had an insulin reaction.

If the blood sugar level drops too low, generally less than 50 mg. per cent (although this varies from person to person), symptoms of insulin reaction or hypoglycemia may occur. Early symptoms are hunger, nausea, trembling, weakness, sweating, confusion, or tingling of the mouth and fingers. If treatment is delayed, or in severe reactions, other symptoms such as headache, confusion, drowsiness or unconsciousness may occur. Hypoglycemia occurs most often in patients who use insulin, but it can also result during use of oral blood-sugar-lowering tablets. Anything that lowers the blood sugar level can cause such a reaction. Many nondiabetics experience mild episodes of hypoglycemia as an entirely normal phenomenon. Consider, for example, the office worker who skips breakfast and late in the morning may have a dull headache. This could mean his blood glucose is lower than normal. Since the symptoms are not severe, episodes of this type are most often ignored. Even without food his symptoms do not become worse, because the nondiabetic does not secrete insulin in the presence of low blood glucose. Likewise, the nondiabetic school child who eats little lunch may be irritable by late afternoon; the traditional cookies and milk late in the afternoon resolve that situation.

LOW BLOOD SUGAR RESULTS FROM:
1. too LITTLE (or no) food
2. too MUCH exercise, without extra food
3. too MUCH insulin

YOU MAY FEEL:
1. shaky
2. sweaty
3. hungry
4. weak
5. dizzy
6. confused

and your urine sugar test would usually be NEGATIVE. YOU SHOULD TAKE:
1. orange juice, or
2. Coke or any other sweetened soda (NOT dietetic), or
3. two lumps of sugar, or
4. several Life Savers or Charms

What causes the symptoms of reaction? When the blood sugar level drops precipitously, epinephrine (adrenaline) is released as part of the body's normal alarm system. This brings stored glucose into the bloodstream, and these epinephrine-related symptoms are usually transient if treated promptly.

If the low blood sugar level is prolonged, the patient may become increasingly confused or sometimes hyperactive to the point of convulsive seizures. Headaches and other central nervous system symptoms are common when the brain receives too little glucose (although it always gets first choice of available body sugar). Sometimes the patient may lose con-

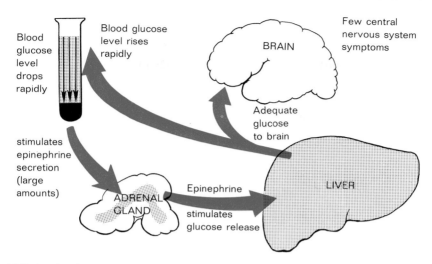

FIG. 23. Insulin reaction due to regular, rapid-acting insulin. The blood glucose level drops rapidly, which causes the release of much epinephrine (adrenaline) from the adrenal gland. The effect of the epinephrine is to mobilize glucose from storage areas in the body, such as the liver. This often corrects the situation. The symptoms that the patient experiences, such as sweating, nervousness, and anxiety, result from the effects of the epinephrine.

sciousness, but this is not common in most patients. Some of the possible symptoms of hypoglycemia due to rapid-acting insulin are shown in Figure 23. Of course, the onset of hypoglycemia can be so mild that it is not easily recognized (reactions without warning). On the other hand, prolonged low blood sugar levels may cause impaired judgment, emotional upset, loss of control, and certainly embarrassment (*Fig. 24*).

The diagnosis of insulin reaction is easy if suspected. Hypoglycemic reactions often tend to be brief when due to rapid (clear) insulin, but they may be persistent or recur when due to long-acting insulin or oral agents. Reactions tend to occur just before a meal is due or when the insulin has its peak effect, especially long after meals. It is important to know the time of peak action and the duration of the insulin or oral agent being used. Reactions before lunch are usually due to rapidly acting regular (clear) insulin, the dose of which is often guided by the pre-lunch urine test. Caution must be used in acting too vigorously to correct these elevated pre-lunch

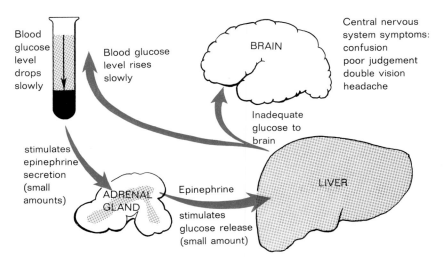

FIG. 24. Insulin reaction due to long-acting insulin. If the blood glucose level drops slowly or for a prolonged period of time, the adrenal gland releases less epinephrine (adrenaline) than occurs with rapid hypoglycemia. Therefore, the amount of glucose released from the body's storage areas is less, and the blood glucose level returns to normal more slowly. The patient experiences fewer symptoms due to the effects of epinephrine, but more symptoms related to the central nervous system, such as confusion, double vision, headache, poor judgement, and even unconsciousness in severely prolonged hypoglycemia.

urine tests with large doses of clear insulin. Sometimes large doses of clear insulin have a prolonged action, and can cause reactions in midafternoon. Another means of combating the high pre-lunch urine test is to adjust the diet.

The intermediate-acting insulins (NPH and Lente) most often cause reactions in the late afternoon or just before the evening meal, and dosage should be adjusted by testing the urine at that time. NPH or Lente insulin taken in the evening can cause reactions during the night or early the next morning.

There is always a reason for an insulin reaction. Sometimes patients continue to use the same dosage of insulin in the spring and summer months, even though the days are longer and they are more active. Doctors note a springtime phenomenon of seemingly epidemic insulin reactions. These patients should counterbalance their increased activity with insulin or diet adjustment as needed. Conversely, in the autumn, some people revert to a limited activity schedule and the urine tests may be elevated. In northern latitudes, with shorter days, early darkness and less activity, it is often necessary to increase the insulin dose.

Differing Patterns of Reaction. A most confusing thing about insulin reactions is how differently they may occur in different people. Patients react differently to the same level of blood sugar. Many persons have obvious symptoms when the blood sugar level drops to 40 mg. per cent, but a certain few may remain quite alert and show no unusual behavior with blood sugar levels as low as 20 mg. per cent. Some persons, while unable to do involved work, can perform automatic, habitual tasks quite well during an insulin reaction. Sometimes a patient seems to be struggling for words; struggling speech is one of the earliest signs of reaction. The patient may deny that anything unusual has occurred, and when he is finally persuaded to drink some orange juice, wonders how he got to the doctor's office. In some, a Jekyll-and-Hyde personality surfaces. The quiet person may become belligerent, or the noisy person thoughtful. Mothers often recognize a low blood sugar level when a usually peaceful child becomes hyperactive or sometimes irrational. Even experienced physicians are caught unawares. One day at the Joslin Clinic, a child was rambunctious, crying and refused to permit his blood to be drawn for testing. Cajoling, threatening, or reasoning with him were equally ineffective. Dr. Elliott P. Joslin noticed this and tried unsuccessfully to convince the child to permit the test. He then asked whether the child was usually afraid of having blood drawn. The mother replied that this was most unusual, and ordinarily the child did not object. Dr. Joslin gave the youngster a small glass of ginger ale, after which the mood change was striking. The child cooperated and it was obvious that his low blood sugar level had changed his usual behavior pattern.

Some persons in insulin reaction behave as though they were intoxicated. They are confused, unstable and erratic in their behavior. One reason for diabetics to abstain from drinking alcohol and driving is that if they have a hypoglycemic reaction and there is an odor of alcohol on their breath, they may be accused of being intoxicated and might even suffer arrest.

In severe low blood sugar episodes, especially those lasting for any prolonged period, unconsciousness may occur. One-sided weakness is sometimes observed and the patient may appear to have suffered a cerebral hemorrhage or "stroke." Fortunately these symptoms are often short in duration with proper treatment.

Diabetics who have hypoglycemia are often stubbornly reluctant to accept treatment; persons attempting to treat the patient often find this behavior difficult to understand. This behavior is part of the reaction itself. When the blood sugar level is low, the brain functions may be affected, and ingenuity may be needed in persuading the patient to accept necessary treatment.

Prevention.   Diabetics should be trained to avoid sudden changes in diet, insulin or exercise and to take their between-meal snacks whether they feel the need or not. Before indulging in vigorous exercise, they should eat extra slow-acting carbohydrates, such as crackers, milk or bread, because the glucose contained in orange juice and ginger ale, although effective, is utilized rapidly. Small amounts of carbohydrate taken every one or two hours during the exercise period are useful. Sometimes, during strenuous exercise, it may be necessary to eat concentrated sweets. *This is an obvious exception to the basic diet rule of avoiding concentrated sweets.*

Prevention is the best form of treatment. If a golfer plans on playing 36 holes of golf, or a student expects to spend a day mountain-climbing, it would probably be wise for each to lower the insulin dose as well as to increase the diet.

Treatment.   *If the patient is conscious,* the simplest, fastest-acting, sweet drink or food available should be taken. Allow 10 to 15 minutes for the sugar to be effective and repeat the same treatment if no improvement is seen. Commonly available drinks are orange juice and regular ginger ale (*not* low-calorie). Other effective choices are two lumps of sugar, a half dozen Life Savers or Charms, two teaspoons of concentrated sugar (as in corn syrup, honey, or Coca Cola syrup), or any sweet available. "Instant Glucose"* is a highly concentrated and rapidly absorbable jell-like form of glucose that is available in a collapsible tube. It is useful for emergencies.

In this day and age, there is little excuse for permitting severe insulin reactions. Almost any gasoline station has carbonated drinks containing sugar available. Patients should carry sweets in their cars or on their persons and keep a supply in their desks at work. Supplies should be checked from time to time, however. One patient who suffered a severe reaction was reprimanded by his physician for not having some candy in the glove compartment of his car. The patient replied that he did have some, but a night or two before the reaction, his young son had found the candy.

The treatment of an unconscious patient poses problems, because liquids should not be force-fed; the patient may aspirate liquid into the trachea (windpipe), thus causing lung complications. Unconscious patients may be treated with injections of glucagon or taken immediately to the physician or hospital emergency room for intravenous glucose.

GLUCAGON.   Like insulin, glucagon is a pancreatic hormone. While insulin is made by the beta cells of the islets of Langerhans, glucagon is the product of the alpha cells. Because it is a chain of protein amino acids, it too must be injected. If the patient is unconscious, glucagon administration must be the responsibility of some member of the family. Glucagon is effective in the treatment of severe hypoglycemia because it releases the stored glycogen from the liver and helps to convert it into glucose in the blood. This temporarily raises the blood sugar level to the point where the unconscious patient will usually awaken and be able to take other nourishment.

Obviously, every diabetic who uses insulin, especially those with juvenile-onset or unstable diabetes, must have glu-

---

*"Instant Glucose" is available from the Diabetes Association of Greater Cleveland (Ohio), 2022 Lee Road, Cleveland, Ohio 44118. It contains 25 grams of carbohydrate. A similar product, Reactose, is made by C.R. Canfield & Co., 2744 Lyndale Avenue S., Minneapolis, Minnesota 55408. Some teaching nurses recommend using small tubes of decorative cake icing, which are available in grocery stores or supermarkets. This icing is sweet and has the consistency of toothpaste.

cagon available for an emergency, and some member of the family should be knowledgeable about its use. Glucagon is injected in the same way as insulin. Ordinarily, the patient will be aroused in five to ten minutes. If there is no response, a second injection may be given. If the response is *still insufficient,* more intensive treatment is indicated and the patient should be taken at once to a hospital emergency room or doctor's office.

Glucagon is available through Eli Lilly and Company in a kit that contains two ampules. One ampule contains 1 mg. of glucagon as a white powder; the other, 1 cc. of sterile solution for preparing the injection. The procedure is simple enough. The tops of both ampules are wiped with alcohol (just as the top of an insulin bottle). Using the insulin syringe and needle, withdraw all of the diluting solution and inject it into the ampule of glucagon powder. Then shake this ampule to dissolve all the powder, and withdraw all of the resulting solution into the syringe. This solution is injected under the patient's skin exactly like insulin. (Epinephrine injection, used for the same purpose before glucagon was developed, is not quite as effective.) The glucagon kit is available by prescription.

The patient who does not respond to glucagon should be rushed to his physician's office or the nearest hospital emergency room for more intensive treatment. Intravenous infusion of a 50% glucose solution will bring about rapid and complete recovery in almost every instance, even with severe insulin reaction. When the patient recovers, it is important to reconstruct the events to determine the reason for the reaction. Often this will turn out to be a delayed or skipped meal. Obviously, steps must be taken to avoid a recurrence.

Are Insulin Reactions Harmful?   Mild hypoglycemic reactions may be the hallmark of good regulation, not because they are desirable, but because it is difficult to fine-tune patients with present-day methods of treatment. Many patients have an exaggerated and unwarranted fear of an insulin reaction. This relates not only to the discomforts encountered during a reaction, but to a fear that repeated bouts of hypoglycemia may result in permanent brain damage. The possibility of lasting damage from minor hypoglycemia is very remote. A calamity might follow a very severe reaction involving unconsciousness for a prolonged period, but this is rare. Insulin reactions are nearly always preventable and presently treatable. However, they can, cause difficulty indirectly, as in the case of an automobile accident caused by hypoglycemia in a patient while driving. The diabetic must be careful to risk neither his life nor that of others. Increasingly, regulations are becoming stricter regarding the driving privilege, and the loss of a driver's license is a real threat. Likewise, the danger of accidents on the job due to hypoglycemia is a real one to life, limb and equipment.

Other Conditions Causing Hypoglycemia. "Reactive hypoglycemia" is a condition that is receiving a lot of attention. It results from the excessive release of insulin in nondiabetics following stimulation by elevated levels of blood glucose. The symptoms are the same as in insulin reaction. Although this condition can occur, it is overdiagnosed.

Tumors of the pancreatic beta cells may also cause hypoglycemia through excessive secretion of insulin. This does not have any relationship to diabetes. Fortunately, this condition is rare, diagnosable and curable.

presbyopia (blurred vision)

Early in the insulin treatment of previously uncontrolled diabetes, many patients undergo an alarming phenomenon. As their diabetes comes under control, their vision starts to blur. This blurring (presbyopia) is not consistent, but things appear to be out of focus. Patients, already worried about their diabetes and having heard of eye problems in diabetes, are thoroughly frightened. This experience is usually short-lived, lasting several days to weeks, and has no relationship to retinal damage or permanent impairment of vision. Because the diabetes had been uncontrolled for some period of time, the patient lost considerable amounts of body fluid, including that contained in the eyeball. Since the eyeball is hollow, any loss of fluid changes its shape. This happens so gradually that the diabetic accommodates to it. With good regulation, fluid returns to all areas of the body, including the eyeballs. This return of fluid again changes the eyeball shape, and there is edema of the lens (swelling caused by fluid accumulation). It takes time to adjust to this, and the vision is temporarily like a picture out of focus. The patient should be reassured; the condition is not permanent. It is one reason why eye doctors will not fit glasses until the diabetes has been stable for about three or four weeks; otherwise, a new set of glasses would be required every few days.

allergy to insulin

Although a generalized allergic reaction to insulin is a rare phenomenon, when it does occur it may be quite serious. It usually occurs in people who had been treated with insulin, which was discontinued and later resumed. People can be desensitized by repeated small injections. The patient must be hospitalized for this. The injections are started with very minute doses of insulin, such as 1/1,000 of a unit or less. The amount is doubled until signs of allergy disappear and the patient is presumably desensitized. Much more common is an allergic reaction that causes itching and some redness at the site of injection. This generally disappears, although medication to relieve itching can be helpful.

insulin resistance

Nearly every diabetic at one time or another has some degree of insulin resistance. Most often this is only relative and may be caused by infection, too generous a diet or some similar reason. True insulin resistance has been defined arbitrarily as requiring 200 units of insulin or more daily. Some patients need as many as 500 to 2000 units daily for a period of time. Several years ago, a Joslin Clinic patient required 16,000 units daily before the period of resistance ended. U-5000 insulin (5000 units in 1 cc. or one syringeful) was used. However, such cases are very rare. Usually they are caused by a high response of antibodies to insulin from a foreign species. Some patients develop high levels of antibody response to one type of insulin (beef or pork) as compared to another, so that sometimes the resistance can be lessened by changing the type of insulin. Resistance may occasionally subside spontaneously. In very stubborn cases, it may be necessary to use large doses of insulin to break the resistance.

insulin abscess and infection

Abscesses and infections at the injection site can develop because of careless injection technique. They are always preventable with proper cleanliness and sterile technique. Some abscesses may be small and treatable with antibiotics; others may develop into very large areas that may require surgical treatment.

insulin atrophy

Atrophy is a complication caused by insulin injections, although no one is exactly certain why. It occurs most often in girls and young women and consists of a loss of fatty tissue just beneath the skin at the sites of injections. This results in unsightly hollows. Parents fear that these hollows will appear continually and that all of the body fat will waste away, but this is not true. There is no significance other than cosmetic. The condition often improves spontaneously over a period of many years as the hollows fill in.

One way to allow improvement is to rotate the insulin injection sites and avoid injecting into the same area. Some patients find it satisfactory to inject into the abdominal area, since most people have more abdomen than they need and the disappearance of fat here might be welcome. High on the thighs used to be a preferred place for injections because presumably these areas were reasonably hidden from public view; this is no longer true, since modern dress leaves little out of sight. A more hopeful note is the fact that the new "single-peak" insulin, a more highly purified insulin, has been used in recent years. This has apparently reduced the occurrence of atrophy. In rare cases when the areas of atrophy are extensive, insulin of extraordinary purity, a monocomponent insulin, may be used. These preparations are not ordinarily available.

Taking advantage of the fact that insulin is lipogenic (encourages fat production) when used locally, the atrophied areas often fill in if the insulin is injected consistently into the sides and depths of the atrophic area.

insulin hypertrophy

This is another complication of insulin injection, with just the opposite effect of atrophy. Tissue sometimes builds up in the areas of injection, usually on the thighs. This is called *hypertrophy*. Although worrisome to the patient, it is harmless.

insulin edema

This condition sometimes occurs in young diabetics starting treatment with insulin. It is found more often in girls and generally is characterized by puffiness, caused by fluid accumulation, occurring around the ankles and also in other areas of the body. Although the fluid amounts are not large, the appearance of such fluid frightens the new diabetic. It is rarely severe enough to require more than reassurance, although sometimes diuretic (fluid-removing) drugs may be used temporarily.

the "Somogyi effect" (rebound)

This is hyperglycemia (high blood glucose) resulting from hypoglycemia (low blood glucose). It can occur when the blood glucose level falls to below normal levels (as in prolonged insulin reaction) and the body tries to compensate by releasing into the blood glucose from the body storage depots. This release of glucose often is not rapid enough. The liver sometimes releases too much glucose producing elevated blood and urine glucose levels. There is no positive pattern to these "rebounds" but they can occur 6 to 12 hours after several strongly positive tests for sugar. Certainly every insulin reaction is not followed by this manifestation. The danger lies in responding to elevated blood glucose tests with too much insulin. The moral is to watch a series of tests rather than to overtreat in either direction. This "Somogyi effect", while not uncommon, is overemphasized as a cause for poor control of diabetes, when the reasons are much simpler and more apparent.

ketoacidosis

At the other end of the spectrum is the complication that most threatens the diabetic—high blood sugar level and its end result, diabetic ketoacidosis or coma. This can occur at any point in the life of the insulin-requiring diabetic. Prior to the discovery of insulin in 1921, nearly half the diabetic deaths in the New England Deaconess Hospital in Boston were due to diabetic coma. At present the death rate is about 1% of those who are admitted with this diagnosis.

> HIGH BLOOD SUGAR RESULTS FROM:
> 1. too MUCH food
> 2. too LITTLE exercise
> 3. too LITTLE insulin
> 4. illness
>
> YOU MAY:
> 1. be THIRSTY
> 2. URINATE frequently
> 3. LOSE weight
> 4. be very TIRED
>
> and your urine sugar test would be POSITIVE
>
> YOU SHOULD:
> 1. test urine for ACETONE
> 2. CALL the DOCTOR
> 3. INCREASE INSULIN DOSE

As the blood sugar levels increase because of the lack of insulin, the body loses tremendous amounts of fluid. The patient becomes dehydrated and because of the insulin lack, a vicious cycle takes place. The body breaks down fats in an attempt to get fuel. Ketone bodies are the end products of improper fat breakdown and these accumulate in the blood and spill over into the urine, where they are recognized as ketonuria. The patient becomes more dehydrated and an acid condition of the blood develops. In extreme cases or when sufficient insulin or fluids are not given soon enough, coma and unconsciousness occur. This complication is always pre- ventable and, in this day, treatable. However, speed is the essence of treatment. This is an emergency as grave as any that a diabetic can face. It is every bit as much of an emergency as acute appendicitis, and more complicated to treat.

Causes. Except in those cases that coincide with the discovery of diabetes, the cause of ketoacidosis can almost always be attributed to one or more precipitating factors. All of these factors lead, in one way or another, to a deficit of needed insulin. The pattern often starts with neglect of diet and other routines, especially vigilance in routine blood testing. It is not likely that poor diet alone ever pushed anyone into ketoacidosis, but accompanying this pattern may be a general neglect of urine testing, and this increasingly poor treatment escalates already high blood sugar levels. At this point it is not difficult for an infection, especially one accompanied by fever, to make insulin less effective. The demand for more insulin is not met because the patient is not aware as yet that the diabetes is severely out of control. The *coup de grace* often takes place when, because of illness and not eating, the patient does not take the usual insulin dose. This makes acidosis almost certain because at that time the patient usually needs more insulin in addition to his usual dose.

Symptoms. The onset of diabetic acidosis leading to coma, in contrast to that of insulin reaction, is gradual. Usually urine sugar and acetone tests are poor over a period of days before the full picture appears. In the juvenile or unstable diabetic, however, coma can develop in 12 to 24 hours (although still with time to avoid the disaster!). At first, the symptoms are often those of untreated diabetes—dry mouth, thirst and excessive urination. Nausea and vomiting are usually present and abdominal pain is frequently found. Later findings may be deep and labored breathing (called Kussmaul respiration), flushed features, dryness, and a general feeling of acute illness that gives way to drowsiness and finally coma. The breath has a sweetish acetone odor. Although the word "coma" implies total loss of unconsciousness, the patient may not be completely unconscious but rather disoriented and increasingly stuporous.

Treatment. Fullblown diabetic acidosis or coma requires emergency medical care in a hospital. *Enough* insulin, not surprisingly, is the foundation of treatment, regardless of the dose needed. The usual initial dose may range from 6 to 200 units of clear, rapidly acting insulin. Sometimes insulin is given intravenously for faster action. The dose for small children is considerably smaller than that for adults. In subsequent hours, insulin doses are guided by the level of blood sugar and by the levels of carbon dioxide and acetone in the blood. Recent studies seem to favor steady infusion of small amounts of insulin.

ONE OF THE MOST COMMON MISTAKES MADE BY DIABETICS IS THE NEGLECT TO TAKE INSULIN ON DAYS THEY ARE ILL. In spite of the fact that they are eating less, insulin may be less effective. They might need MORE insulin, not less.

The other vital treatment is replacement of body fluid intravenously to correct the intense dehydration that accompanies acidosis. Potassium, lost because of excessive urination, must be replaced and shock treated. Later, liquids by mouth, at first in tiny amounts, are started when tolerated. By the second day, the patient is usually able to take small amounts of food, and when the chemical constituents of the blood are close to normal, the usual program of insulin and diet is resumed. Usually several more days of diabetes regulation follow to facilitate the patient's return to normal.

Prevention. Although today diabetic coma is not the dreaded nightmare that it was in the pre-insulin era, it is still a very serious complication. With coma, as with insulin reaction, prevention is the keynote, and today, with the possible exception of cases occurring at the onset of diabetes, ketoacidosis can nearly always be avoided. It is here that the education of the diabetic and his family is most important. The inadequately trained patient may bumble along from day to day under ordinary circumstances with no severe penalties until confronted by illness, infection or inadequate insulin. *Always take your usual daily dose of insulin—do not omit it when feeling ill.* Remember that, during illness, the liver is releasing glucose *even when one is unable to eat,* resulting in a need for insulin. In fact, the amount of insulin needed during illness may far exceed the usual daily dose. Regardless of the circumstances, persistent poor urine tests mean lack of insulin. You should always:

1. Check the urine for sugar daily as directed by your physician. Two or three times daily is minimal. Four times is ideal.
2. Use all available means (diet, exercise, insulin) to keep the urine as sugar-free as possible.
3. Test for acetone (ketones) if the urine sugar test is strongly positive.
4. During an infection, increase the dose of insulin if the urine tests are strongly positive.
5. Take additional insulin as your doctor may order.
6. Treat all illnesses as possible impending coma and follow sick-day rules.

SICK-DAY RULES. There are times in life when emergency rules supersede all other regulations. The possibility of acidosis or coma developing is one of these emergencies. (See "Sick Day Rules" in Appendix 7.) Certainly the physician should be called as soon as possible for advice. The rules as given are subject to considerable variation, and every patient should know what his own doctor wants him to do.

differences between high and low blood sugar levels

Since ketoacidosis and insulin reaction are such serious complications, it is important to be able to differentiate between them and to start appropriate treatment as early as possible. The guidelines for this are shown in Table 20. In most situations, these conditions are not difficult to differentiate from one another—the nature of the onset of symptoms is important. A fast change from normal is usually a sign of low blood sugar. Initially, if a patient is conscious, give sugar by mouth, preferably in a liquid form. If the patient cannot swallow, give an injection of glucagon. When in doubt, treat as if the patient is having an insulin reaction, *unless evidence of ketoacidosis appears.*

TABLE 20. Differentiating Between Insulin Reaction and Hyperglycemia and Possible Ketoacidosis.

Hypoglycemic Reaction		Hyperglycemia and Impending Coma
Sudden	ONSET	Slow
Moist skin	APPEARANCE	Dry skin
Nervous, some-times confused	ACTIONS	Drowsy and sometimes stuporous
Sweating Shaking Hungry Weak	SYMPTOMS	Nausea Vomiting Dehydrated Sweetish breath (acetone)
Low	BLOOD SUGAR	High to very high
None, but possibly present if bladder not emptied for a long period	URINE SUGAR	+ + + +
None	URINE ACETONE	+ + + +

summary

The major acute complications of diabetes, insulin reaction and ketoacidosis, are not only treatable but usually preventable. Success in avoiding these conditions, which can occur early or late in the course of diabetes, depends on the patient's knowledge of diabetes and its control. Diabetes should be respected but not feared. Education is vital in avoiding these pitfalls.

9

Long-Term
Complications

9

The expression "long-term complications" is a definition chosen to separate these late problems from those discussed earlier. It means that while the "acute" complications discussed in the previous section can occur anytime after diabetes is found, the problems presented here are not likely to occur, if indeed they ever will, until the diabetes has been present for some years. Many persons with diabetes now live 50 years or longer free from some significant difficulties. On the other hand, while the "acute" complications can nearly all be averted, the possibility of avoiding long-term changes is less certain. It may be easy to generalize about "good regulation" of diabetes being better for patients, but it is not easy to show that specific levels of blood sugar above or below a certain point will definitely prevent these problems. However, some of these complications are more easily avoidable than others.

the eyes

The possibility of damage to the eyes or vision causes the greatest fear among diabetics. It is true that diabetes is a leading cause of blindness in the United States. It is equally true that relatively few diabetics become completely blind, possibly not more than 5%. Do these statements seem to conflict? There really is a paradox. Although the latest available U.S. Public Health Service figures state that there are more than 155,000 blind diabetics in the United States, this refers to *legal* blindness and not *total* blindness. A person may be legally blind (20/200 vision or less), and still have enough vision to get around. Although many long-term diabetics may have decreased vision, an amazing number of them have a static condition that does not worsen; some even improve. One problem is that the blind person is highly visible: 50 patients with good vision may be sitting in a clinic waiting room, but the one person without sight is noticed by everyone.

Nonetheless, degenerative eye changes in diabetes is a serious problem. It is estimated that by the year 2000 there will be more than a half-million sightless diabetics if improved methods of prevention or treatment are not found. One reason for the increasingly large numbers of blind diabetics is that diabetics now live long enough to develop many complications that were relatively unknown when the life span of a person with diabetes was much shorter.

Eye Structure.   The eye is a strange and wonderful instrument. Essentially it is like a hollow pingpong ball filled with a clear fluid called vitreous (*Fig. 25*). Next to the vitreous is the retina, which is the delicate nervous membrane that responds to visual stimuli. The retina is connected to the optic nerve by nerve fibers. The human optic nerve has about 1,200,000 individual nerve fibers, which are most densely packed in the

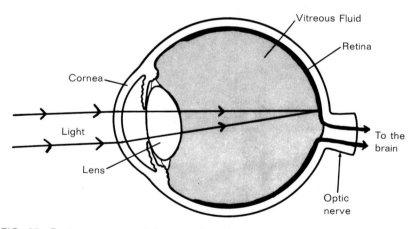

FIG. 25. Basic structure of the eye (profile view). Light passes through the cornea and the lens and is focused on the rear of the eyeball at the layer of the retina. The optic nerve carries the image from the retina to the brain, where it is interpreted. The vitreous is a clear fluid that keeps the eyeball in constant shape. Three areas of potential trouble are (1) clouding of the lens, which is known as *cataract;* (2) increased pressure of the eyeball fluid, which can damage the optic nerve, a condition called *glaucoma;* (3) rupture or hemorrhage of the blood vessels in the retina, a condition called *retinitis* or *diabetic retinopathy.*

center of the nerve that carries images from the middle of the retina. The optic nerve at the back of the eye goes directly to the brain. As the physician looks into the pupil of the eye, he sees a pale, yellow, flat object, much like a pancake, on the back of the eyeball. That is the flat side of the optic nerve facing him. Coming out of all the sides of this optic disc are blood vessels, like the spokes of a wheel (*Fig. 26*). These blood vessels are important because they nourish the eye. The arteries and veins are called retinal vessels. The physician also sees another area close to the optic disc, called the macula, which controls central vision.

Although the eye has often been described as a camera, it is much more complicated than that. It chooses the proper amount of light needed and adjusts its own focal length better than the most perfect camera made. It even protects itself with a lid when necessary. It has a lens in front, very much like the lens in a camera. Any clouding that might occur in the lens itself is called a *cataract*. The fluid going in and out of the eyeball is constantly changing. If something stops the proper drainage of fluid from the eyeball so that the pressure increases, this condition is called *glaucoma*. Inflammation of the outer front covering of the eye, so that it looks red or hemorrhagic, is known as *conjunctivitis*. Damage to the retinal blood vessels so that they break, leak or bleed is known as *hemorrhagic retinitis* (*Fig. 27*). It is this last condition that most threatens vision for many diabetics. Vascular (blood vessel) changes in the eye are fairly common in long-term diabetes, but complete blindness is not nearly as common as supposed. Although about 90% of those who have had diabetes for more than 25 years have some vascular changes, sometimes these are not obvious to the patient and they may not impair vision.

Subconjunctival Hemorrhage. Occasionally a person looks into the mirror and sees a bright red, pie-shaped wedge in the white of the eye. This is frightening but quite harmless. It represents a tiny blood vessel that somehow broke and bled beneath the outside covering. It is not exclusive to diabetics; anyone can have it. It is not a complication of diabetes; if left alone, it usually improves and disappears within a few days.

Glaucoma. Many persons over age 40 are candidates for glaucoma, and persons in that age group should be tested for glaucoma every year or two. The test is simple, quick and

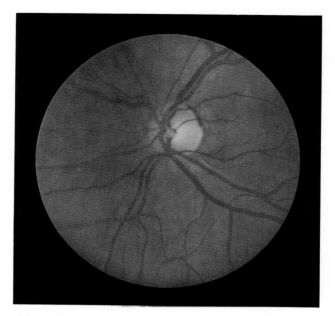

FIG. 26. The fundus of the normal eye. The round disc in the center is the optic nerve. The blood vessels radiate from the center like spokes in a wheel. The thicker ones are veins; the thinner ones, arteries. (From Nover, A. (F.C. Blodi, trans.): The Ocular Fundus. 3rd ed. Philadelphia, Lea & Febiger, 1974.)

painless; it is done with an instrument called a tonometer which measures eyeball pressure. Increased pressure is due to too much fluid in the eye. At first the condition causes no symptoms. As the pressure increases, the symptoms may include visual loss and bright flashes or rings of lights around the eyes. Later there may be eye pain. If left untreated too long, the pressure damage is irreversible. Early the condition is treated with eyedrops that permit the fluid exchange to continue. Sometimes surgery is helpful. The usual forms of glaucoma (increased pressure without hemorrhage) may occur in diabetics as in nondiabetics. Glaucoma resulting from hemorrhage is fortunately unusual.

Cataract. A cataract (clouding of the lens) is one of the commonest eye problems that occurs in older people. The lens must remain transparent if vision is to be normal. If the lens

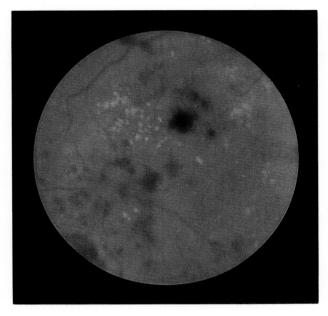

FIG. 27. Diabetic retinopathy, showing numerous hemorrhages and degenerative deposits. (From Nover, A. (F.C. Blodi, trans.): The Ocular Fundus. 3rd ed. Philadelphia, Lea & Febiger, 1974.)

becomes clouded, the transmission of light is blocked. There are two types of cataract. One type is the metabolic cataract, which develops because of the accumulation of the by-products of abnormal metabolism in the lens of the eye. This type of cataract is sometimes found in younger people; before the use of insulin, metabolic cataracts were quite common in diabetics. The most common type of cataract is the so-called senile cataract, frequently found in older people with or without diabetes. Senile cataract seems to occur as part of the normal aging process, although there is some evidence that poor control of diabetes may accelerate the process. Either of these two types of cataract can be treated surgically by removing the lens. New eyeglasses replace the lens.

Diseases of the Retina.   Damage or disease of the retina (retinopathy) is the most serious of all the diabetic complications of the eye. The early changes of diabetic retinopathy start subtly. The small retinal vessels weaken and their supporting basement membranes (the lining of the vessels) become thickened and develop leaks. The vessels themselves become fragile. Recent research has shown that the chemical makeup of this basement membrane is changed in diabetes.

A more obvious change is the microaneurysm, a dilated bulge on the wall of a small vessel, which is pretty much like the bulge on the side of a weakened automobile tire. Such little bulges may leak serum from the blood. A more dangerous type of retinopathy is the formation of many new and very fragile vessels. This process of new vessel formation is called neovascularization; it is proliferative. Major hemorrhages of these fragile vessels can result in the formation of small, dark streaks. If the hemorrhages are large enough or cover a sensitive area, they interfere with vision. They may rupture through the retinal lining into the fluid of the eye, discoloring the vitreous so that vision is blocked. This is known as vitreal hemorrhage.

Happily, many small hemorrhages may be absorbed, and within days or weeks even the vitreal hemorrhage may clear up because the eye fluid is continually being changed. If the new vessels shrink and scar, the visual loss may not become worse. It has been estimated that in about 30% of patients with vessel disease of this type, the visual loss does not necessarily progress but remains static or even improves spontaneously. In one large series of patients whose eyes were observed from the time they first showed some evidence of retinal damage, after 15 years 18% had an increased visual loss but twice as many (36%) were either no worse or actually had improved.

A technique of injecting fluorescein dye into the eye circulation so that the vessels can be outlined gives the physician a precise view of the damage. This, in turn, helps to pinpoint areas suitable for treatment.

Treatment of Damaged Retina. The treatment of diseased retina has improved in recent years. In the past there have been many attempts to treat retinal disease, and most have been useless.

Good control of diabetes has always been considered helpful in preventing retinopathy. Many of those who have lived 20 to 50 years with diabetes without severe forms of eye damage have usually taken better care of their diabetes than those who have severe eye damage after this length of time. However, this factor is difficult to pinpoint in individual cases; some diabetics have retinal changes as early as ten years after the onset of their condition.

REMOVAL OF PITUITARY GLAND. Because anterior pituitary growth hormone increases the severity of diabetes, attempts to improve diabetes and lessen retinopathy were made by destroying the pituitary gland (situated at the base of the brain). This was done by surgical removal, by cutting the stalk of the gland, or by irradiation, using x-rays or implants of radioactive substances to destroy the pituitary. In those whose pituitary was destroyed or removed, the insulin requirement did fall and perhaps 50% of these patients showed regression of the eye damage with consequently stabilized or improved vision. Such neurosurgery, however, is a complex procedure which causes functional loss in the thyroid, adrenals and sex hormone production, so that the patient may require thyroid extract, cortisone and sex hormones indefinitely. He also becomes exquisitely sensitive to small changes in insulin. In a sense, there is an exchange of one abnormal state for several, and the patient becomes an "endocrine cripple." While the success rate of about 50% over a five-year period is not very promising, sight is so precious that many have undergone these difficult procedures, sometimes with good results. The risks are great and although a few medical centers still treat in this fashion, enthusiasm for this therapy has diminished greatly.

PHOTOCOAGULATION (TREATMENT WITH LIGHT). A new and exciting era in the treatment of retinopathy has dawned with the development of photocoagulation techniques. These dramatic new procedures use concentrated light rays from a xenon arc (white light), an argon laser (green light), or a ruby laser (red light). These lights are focused on the retina and coagulate leaking blood vessels (xenon) or, in the case of the ruby laser, emit a beam of pure red light that can be transmitted through blood vessels without harming them. The red light is picked up by the retina, resulting in numerous tiny areas of change. This appears to decrease the demand for blood, so that the delicate and unneeded proliferative vessels tend to regress, reducing the likelihood of further bleeding. The latest laser, the argon (or green laser), can do anything the other methods do but with much more precision. It can directly obliterate bleeding vessels and pinpoint specific areas with great accuracy. "Laser" itself is an acronym (artificial word) derived from the first letters of the words "Light Amplification by Stimulated Emission of Radiation."

These procedures have been developed recently and are being evaluated. They have not yet been used for long periods or in large numbers of patients. However, the outlook is hopeful. In some series of patients it has been reported that the proper use of lasers may have been useful in 50 to 70% of the cases. The xenon arc may damage some good retinal areas, so that while the bleeding may have stopped, the visual field may be smaller. The lasers, on the other hand, even if not effective in some people, rarely do any damage. At this time, photocoagulation is not a cure-all and is not useful in all types of retinopathy. With more experience and possibly better lasers, there may be more help for diabetic eyes in the future. However, the laser therapy seems to be a big improvement over any previous attempts at treatment.

The National Eye Institute of the National Institutes of Health released a report on the preliminary results of the Diabetic Retinopathy Study, which was started in 1971 and involved 15 medical centers. This controlled study reported that extensive "scatter" photocoagulation and treatment of new (undesirable) vessels has been helpful in preventing severe visual loss over a two-year followup period in eyes with proliferating retinopathy. Further observations are obviously necessary.

VITRECTOMY. A new and remarkable procedure has been used recently. A problem with leaking retinal vessels is that, with a large hemorrhage into the vitreous, the eyeball fluid becomes mixed with blood, preventing light from passing through the eye and thus causing blindness. Until now, little could be done because even lasers could not be used if the doctor could not see into the eye. A surgical procedure called vitrectomy uses a remarkable instrument containing a drill and suction. This enters the eyeball, removes the vitreous hemorrhage and replaces it with normal saline. The instrument is removed and the hole sealed. The ophthalmologist can then see into the eye and determine whether lasers might be helpful. Some remarkable results have been obtained, but the use of vitrectomy is still limited and undergoing evaluation. Many special tests are needed to determine retinal function. These include studies with ultrasound and electroretinogram to determine suitable candidates for this procedure.

the kidneys and urinary tract

The kidneys are among the least appreciated and most abused organs of the body. The urinary tract consists of two kidneys located on either side of the backbone. Long slender tubes called ureters carry the urine from the kidneys to the bladder, which acts as a storage reservoir until the urine is released.

The kidneys have a most important function. They filter the waste products from the blood, retaining the important and useful elements for further use. The end products of protein metabolism are nitrogen substances, which are removed by the kidneys and eliminated. The urinary tract often becomes infected in the diabetic, especially in women and in those with poor regulation of diabetes. In the presence of elevated blood sugar levels, the phagocytes (cells that form part of the body's defenses) may be less effective in destroying bacteria, as shown in recent research. Some common conditions resulting in damage to the kidneys are infection, elevated blood pressure, inflammation of the connective tissues and changes in tissues caused by diabetes. Sometimes these disorders are chronic and progressive and result in uremia. Some of the common complications of the urinary tract in diabetes are shown in Figure 28. Many kidney problems are now treatable.

Urinary Tract Infections. The best solution to urinary tract infection is early diagnosis and adequate treatment. Such infections can be suspected from symptoms such as burning or painful urination, frequency of urination, or cloudy or bloody urine. Early mild urinary infections may produce no symptoms and are detected by frequent, periodic microscopic examination of the urinary sediment, and cultures of urine specimens when needed.

Urinary tract infections are treated with sulfonamides and antibiotics, but treatment must be under medical supervision

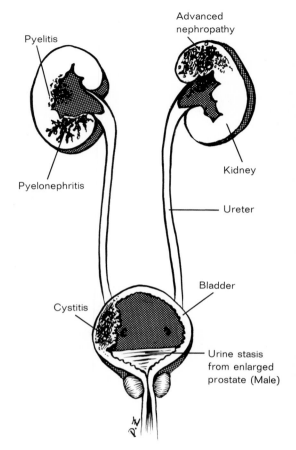

FIG. 28. Common urinary tract complications in diabetes. *Nephropathy* means pathology of the kidney (see text). *Pyelitis* is infection of the pelvis, the area where urine is collected before going down the ureters to the bladder. *Pyelonephritis* is infection of the tubules (which collect the urine), the glomeruli (the little structures that filter the urine from the blood), and the blood vessels. *Cystitis* means inflammation of the bladder, usually as a result of infection. *Urine stasis* means the retention of urine in the bladder owing to obstruction of free urine drainage or bladder atony (see text). The longer urine remains in the bladder, the greater the risk of infection.

because the appropriate antibiotic must be chosen, based on urine culture and sensitivity tests. Treatment must continue until infection is eradicated or it will recur and become chronic.

Diabetic Bladder Dysfunction (Bladder Atony). A problem that occurs infrequently is diabetic bladder atony. The bladder becomes insensitive, overdistended and loses most of its muscle contraction power due to damage to the nerves that control this function. The damage results from diabetic neuropathy and is often associated with other neuropathies as well. This results in incomplete emptying of the bladder and stagnation of urine. Stagnation favors the growth of bacteria and the development of infection. Bladder atony is difficult to treat. Sometimes medicine can be helpful. At other times, surgery is necessary to improve the drainage.

Pathology of the Kidney. Nephropathy is the most serious kidney disorder of diabetes. The word "nephropathy" refers to a combination of three changes that are found together in the kidneys of many people with diabetes of long duration. These changes are infection, sclerosis (hardening of the small kidney arteries) and damage to the glomeruli (filtering apparatus of the kidney). These often progress with the duration of diabetes so that kidney function gradually deteriorates. At first, protein, which usually is saved by the kidneys, starts to appear in the urine in increasing amounts. This protein, in the form of albumin, increases and more of the body's waste products are retained in the blood. In time, water is also retained, which causes swelling (edema). Blood pressure becomes elevated and the classic signs of uremia become more apparent.

The earliest changes are those found with thickening of the basement membranes of the kidney. Some researchers believe that this thickening appears even before the glucose tolerance changes. Increasingly, however, evidence seems to link kidney disease with poor diabetic care. Another important factor is the early recognition and treatment of urinary tract infections.

Treatment of Kidney Disease. In the past, little could be done for people with advanced diabetic nephropathy. Now, modern advances make treatment possible. In advanced cases, it is possible to rid the body of wastes normally excreted by the kidneys with the use of peritoneal dialysis or with the artificial kidney machine. In this method, a machine takes the blood from the patient, removes the impurities, and returns the blood to the patient. However, little can be done to prevent these impurities from being formed. Not all diabetics are suitable candidates for this. If a person has coronary artery disease, peripheral vascular disease, or severe retinopathy, treatment with the artificial kidney may not be useful. Although long-term management of renal failure using the artificial kidney is expensive and not always readily available, the facilities for providing such treatment are increasing and becoming more efficient, even though it may be some time before the need of all patients requiring them is met.

Another means of treating chronic renal failure is renal transplantation. This involves the removal of a healthy kidney, preferably from a near relative of a diabetic or, if such is not available, from some other acceptable donor, and placing it into the diabetic whose own kidneys have stopped functioning. Kidney transplant is a complex and difficult procedure which, while successful in some diabetics, is not yet widely available. Diabetic patients with kidney transplants have not been observed long enough to determine the eventual success of such treatment, but increasing numbers of people are living longer with this form of treatment.

Much is being learned about the choice of patients likely to achieve success with these new methods. Transplantation may prove to be preferable because of the severe limitations that hemodialysis imposes on patients dependent on it. Survival rates are improving, and recent statistics give a one-year kidney survival rate for transplants from related, living donors as 90% or more. Successful transplantation permits the patient to resume nearly normal activities, but patients still require the regular use of drugs to suppress the immunity factors that might cause rejection of the kidney.

In summary, kidney problems begin early and subtly. Many persons have urinary tract infections that are not noticed. In the diabetic, this can have serious consequences. While thickening of the basement membrane cannot always be attributed to poor control of diabetes, there is increasing evidence that such a relationship exists in many cases.

Microscopic urine testing is an important part of the examination of any diabetic. The urine is checked for the presence of pus cells, blood, casts or other evidence of disease, as well as for the usual sugar and albumin levels.

For long-term diabetics with far-advanced kidney damage, treatment is more difficult, but new improved techniques are starting to offer more hope for this group also.

neuropathy (nerve pathology)

Numerous nerve-related problems are loosely lumped under the terms "diabetic neuritis" or "neuropathy." These are among the most puzzling complications of diabetes. This condition is sometimes difficult to diagnose definitely. The symptoms can affect almost any nerve pathway in any part of the body. They can be extremely mild and merely annoying or, on the other hand, very disabling and crippling. While severe neuropathy can be very debilitating, it almost never causes death, unless there are other complications. Diabetic neuropathy is often a diagnosis of exclusion after other conditions have been ruled out. The most common symptoms of neuritis are mild numbness, tingling or pain. There can be sensation loss or severe pain. These symptoms do not respect age or sex, and while any diabetic can have these manifestations, a period of uncontrolled diabetes often but not always precedes the appearance of symptoms. In some adults, these symptoms may lead to the discovery of diabetes. Sometimes the first severe symptoms start after treatment begins but more often, they occur after long duration of diabetes. Fortunately, the symptom of pain often abates in the face of careful treatment of the diabetes. Although neuritis may occur in nearly any nerve, anywhere within the body, certain nerves are affected more frequently than others.

Symptoms of Neuropathy.   Numbness, coldness, tingling, a feeling of walking upon wool, and pain are the most frequent symptoms described by patients. These sensations are most obvious at night on cold, wet, rainy days and in winter. They may be mild or severe, occasional or constant. The skin of the feet, legs and thighs may be so sensitive that the weight of bedclothes is intolerable. Most often the sensory nerves are involved, although the muscle functions can also be affected.

If the symptoms include loss of sensation, foot problems may develop. The patient fails to recognize minor injuries, blisters and trauma. Immediate medical treatment of even the most innocent-looking lesion of the foot is most important.

Amyotrophy (muscle-wasting) is a special form of diabetic neuropathy. It combines extreme sensitivity of the skin of the thighs, pain and tenderness of the thigh muscles, and weakness. Muscle bulk decreases, making it difficult for the person to arise from a chair or to climb stairs. Loss of appetite and subsequent decline of body weight are frequent complaints. With relief of pain, careful treatment of diabetes, and sometimes a preliminary period of nearly absolute bed rest, the condition improves. Muscles may regain their strength, although they may never regain their previous configuration. Recovery is slow.

Occasionally a single nerve that operates a muscle or group of muscles is affected. This type of neuropathy can cause *double vision* if the muscles of eye control are involved. These symptoms continue from three to six weeks. Complete recovery is the rule. The condition may appear more than once in the same person but often different muscles are involved.

Another example of neuropathy is *foot-drop*. The muscles responsible for raising the foot become weakened and the foot slaps with each step. Should the muscles not regain strength, a brace may be worn. However, recovery often takes place.

A relatively less common type of neuropathy is *radicular pain*, which causes an encircling or girdle-type pain in the chest or trunk nerves. It is a sharp, shooting, burning pain that is constant, excruciating, and sometimes defies definition. It usually gradually disappears.

The stomach, small bowel, large bowel and urinary bladder empty their contents by a series of rhythmic contractions of the muscles within their walls. When the nerves that operate these muscles become "neuropathic" delay in the contractions takes place. The patient experiences fullness, bloating, vomiting of undigested food, infrequent but voluminous urination and constipation. Sometimes medication that stimulates smooth muscle function is helpful.

Neuritis can also cause low blood pressure when a patient rises. This is also called *orthostatic hypotension.*

Impotence, the loss of the ability to have erections and

ejaculations, may occur in men after long periods of diabetes. This is thought to be a form of neuropathy.

A rare and little understood form of diabetic neuropathy involves changes in the small bones of the foot. The condition is relatively painless but the bone structure may be injured unless walking is monitored during the acute period. This condition is called *Charcot joint.*

All forms of neuropathy are troublesome to patients and a few may be temporarily disabling. Rarely are they permanent. Most symptoms disappear completely or improve. Nevertheless, in spite of this reassurance, occasionally cases occur that would try the patience of Job. Sometimes the lack of response to medication depresses the patient and frustrates the physician.

Cause of Neuropathy.   The cause of neuropathy is not known. In the past it has been blamed on insufficient nutrition or destruction of the nerves, thrombosis (plugging) of the vessels leading to the nerves, insufficient vitamins and many other factors. The precise reason is not yet known, but while neuropathy remains an enigma, recent research findings have described a "polyol pathway." In persons with persistently high blood sugar levels, metabolic degradation products result in the formation of a substance known as sorbitol, which is deposited in the nerve sheaths and other tissues. These studies may give a more definite answer concerning the onset of neuritis.

Treatment.   Any condition as poorly understood as neuropathy seems to have many treatments, none of which are specific and many of which are not universally effective. Some patients respond to better diabetic care. Others are helped by heat or bed rest. Certain complications, such as fall in blood pressure on arising or lack of sufficient muscle tone, may require special treatment. If the polyol pathway theory is true, sufficient insulin should be available as much of the time as possible to keep the blood sugar levels close to normal. Meanwhile, various analgesic compounds are used, hopefully until the day when either the patient overcomes the neuritis or it remits of its own accord.

cardiovascular complications

The effect of diabetes on cardiovascular disease is difficult to prove. In any event, arteriosclerotic heart disease is the greatest single cause of death in the United States. Certainly some of the more than half million people who die yearly from this condition also have diabetes. In some studies, a third to a half of the patients with a recent heart attack have had an abnormal glucose tolerance test, at least temporarily. It is difficult to determine which disorder came first.

In a population sample study in Tecumeh, Michigan, members of the study group were given glucose tolerance tests, and the highest 22% were considered diabetic. The coronary disease rate was doubled in those with diabetes.

Although all of the factors correlating heart disease with diabetes are not known, myocardial infarction is the chief cause of death in persons with onset of diabetes after age 30. Many diabetics have less obvious coronary symptoms than nondiabetics, but they require more intensive medical care. In an 18-year follow-up of the Framingham Heart Disease and Epidemiological Study, persons with diabetes had at least a doubled incidence of cardiovascular episodes. It is believed that the more the risk factors are eliminated, the less the likelihood of cardiac disease. Elevated blood pressure, smoking and overweight are among the poor risk factors. Among the factors protecting the cardiac system are normal weight and blood pressure, and normal blood levels of fat and sugar.

In addition to improved medical care for all cardiac patients, improved surgical treatment, such as the coronary "by-pass" operation, is available for some types of coronary heart disease. The most useful measure for diabetics is greater vigilance to prevent heart disease.

Blood Vessel Changes. Thickening of parts of the walls of the large blood vessels is believed to be associated with diabetes. This is already a phenomenon of aging and it is adversely influenced by diabetes. Insulin deficiency, reflected by elevated blood sugar levels, may bring about changes in the metabolism of vascular tissue. Increased blood levels of lipids also are harmful. Good diabetic care and medications that lower the blood lipid level as well as decreased intake of fats in the diet may be helpful.

The smaller blood vessels of the eyes and kidneys are more susceptible to metabolic disorders in diabetes (see pp. 168 and 173). Early in its course, this microangiopathy (small blood vessel disease) may be reversible.

infections

It is true that diabetics may have more infections than nondiabetics. However, the old adage that "diabetics don't heal as well as others" is not necessarily true. For example, young people with excellent circulation and reasonably good control of diabetes heal just as rapidly as anyone else. The healing problem occurs more often in older persons with poor circulation in the feet and legs and in those whose diabetes is poorly controlled.

Twenty or thirty years ago, the bane of the diabetic and a frequent cause of death was carbuncles. These are rarely seen now. This is true of many infections that were common before the discovery of antibiotics and the better use of insulin. However, infections are still a hazard to the unwary diabetic. For years it was thought that high levels of blood sugar provided a better breeding area for bacteria, but this was not confirmed. Probably, in the presence of infection, more glucagon is released and more insulin is required. Now it has been shown that the natural body defense against infection may be defective in poorly regulated diabetes. Phagocytes (the white cells that help to fight infection) appear to be much less effective in uncontrolled diabetes. However, their activity is restored to normal with good treatment. In an editorial, the *British Medical Journal* stated, "Perhaps the injunction for diabetics should be to disinhibit the phagocytes by effectively lowering blood sugar."

the foot

The diabetic's foot may be his "Achilles' heel." The feet of diabetics are particularly vulnerable to problems for several reasons (*Fig. 29*): (1) the circulation is decreased in older persons, especially where the blood vessels become narrow at the lower end of the foot; (2) in persons with diabetes, the

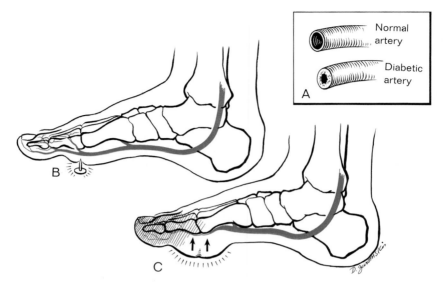

FIG. 29. Foot complications are often caused by diminished blood supply.
(A) The thickened artery of the long-term diabetic permits less blood to circulate
than a normal artery. (B) An injury that causes inflammation requires an even
greater blood supply, which is often unavailable. (C) The infected foot swells,
compressing the arteries and thereby further diminishing the blood supply.

degree of narrowing may be even greater; (3) in diabetes,
sensation may be decreased because of neuropathy. These
factors, coupled with an increased tendency to develop infection in poorly treated diabetes, provide a background for impending trouble.

Any precipitating infection or mechanical impediment,
such as an ingrown toenail, an infected callus or corn, trauma,
untreated athlete's foot or a tight shoe, may damage the tissue
and serve as a portal for infection. As the infection spreads,
inflammation and swelling occur, requiring a greater blood
supply which is not available. A chain of events takes place in
which one thing makes another worse. The infection spreads,
aided by inadequate circulation. The patient has diminished
pain sensation and continues to walk on the injured part, so
the foot crisis deepens.

The most common lesions are corns, calluses (especially
on the toes and soles of the feet), ingrown toenails, fungus

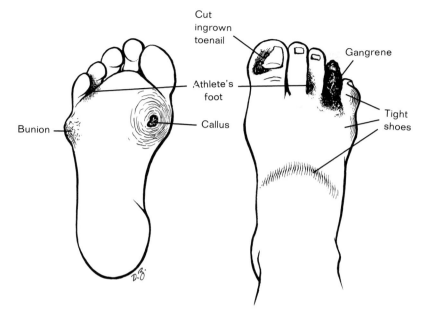

FIG. 30. Some common foot problems in diabetics caused by improper care.

infection (athlete's foot), ulcers caused by pressure—indeed injuries or infections of any kind. Then, of course, deformities due to neuropathic changes may exist. Some of these problems are shown in Figure 30.

Principles of Good Foot Care.   In general, three basic considerations underlie all good foot care:
1. Give the foot good preventive care.
2. Avoid injury to the foot.
3. Wear well-fitted shoes.

SKIN CARE.   Most of the common foot problems involve the skin. In general, it is a good idea to apply a lotion containing lanolin nightly to the feet. However, the web spaces should not be saturated with lotions, which may macerate the skin. When the skin is too moist, apply talcum or baby powder daily to absorb the moisture. If the skin is too dry, apply lotion more frequently. Never nick the skin with scissors or sharp instruments. The skin of the feet should be washed daily, never soaked.

NAIL CARE.   It is a good rule never to cut nails but only to file them down. If the nails are extra thick owing to fungal infections or previous injury, they should be trimmed by a podiatrist.

SOME PHARMACY ITEMS for good foot care are:

Emery boards for filing nails.

pHisoHex, an antibacterial, soapless skin cleanser, is useful for washing any suspected infected area.

ST-37, a mild but effective antiseptic.

A lanolin product or a water-attracting agent for moistening dry feet.

A nonallergenic tape that will not pull off skin or irritate it.

Bacitracin ointment for infected areas. This must be obtained by prescription.

INJURY can result from a number of different causes.

1. Heat (this includes sunburn, electric heating pads, hot or warm water bottles, walking barefoot on a hot pavement).
2. Cold and frostbite.
3. Pressure from shoes, wrinkled stockings or sandal straps.
4. Chemicals and strong patent medicines (for example, alcohol or iodine).
5. Adhesive tape.

General first-aid measures include the following:

1. Always rest an injured or infected foot. The foot does not have to be elevated, but needs only to be extended straight on a hassock, bed or lounge-type chair.
2. Use only mild cleansing agents and antiseptics. Never use iodine, Lysol or colored agents. Dry after using soap. Use nonallergenic tape if a dressing must be applied (paper tape is good).
3. Limit all dressings to simple, sterile "cling" bandages. These should be loosely applied when the foot is at rest.
4. Antibiotic ointments may be used sparingly.

5. Do not be deceived by the absence of pain in an affected foot. Spreading infection can go unnoticed when normal sensation is impaired by neuropathy.

ILL-FITTED SHOES.   Unfortunately, foot types are often not considered in the average measurements of shoe size. A 10B size does not consider problems of the instep, a narrow heel, or even fifth toe deformity. A podiatrist should be consulted for the proper fitting of shoes for diabetics.

Athlete's Foot.   Athlete's foot (dermatophytosis) is a common fungus infection of the feet. It may remain scaly, dry and unnoticed, or it may break out as an inflamed area with broken skin, often between the toes. Feet that perspire heavily seem to be more susceptible to this infection. The fungus can be acquired in locker rooms or from bathroom floors.

Athlete's foot is serious in the diabetic because of its potential for further infection. The treatment of athlete's foot includes the following measures:

1. Treat *both* the skin area involved and the insides of shoes. Wet shoes or sneakers are a source of re-infection.
2. Antifungal ointment (Desenex and Tinactin are commonly used medications) must be used on the affected skin areas for an extended period of time. Using antifungal powder in shoes as a general preventative at least twice a week after the acute infection has ended is a good practice.
3. Wear clogs in the bathroom or shower.
4. Keep feet dry with regular powder, especially when feet are likely to perspire profusely.

Prevention.   The tragedy is that so many foot problems are preventable. In one year in the New England Deaconess Hospital, 417 of about 5000 diabetic patients admitted for care also had foot problems. These 417 people remained in the hospital for a total of 10,742 days, a much longer average stay than that of other patients. If the average cost per hospital day was $100 at that time, this means that more than one million dollars was spent on foot care in one year in only one hospital. This did not include medical or surgical costs and did not take into consideration the pain, time lost from work, or the impact of illness on the rest of the patients' families. In a recent study of hospitalized, patients with foot disorders, it was estimated that about one-third of these disorders could have been prevented, while another third might have been prevented.

Many patients, particularly older persons, don't examine their feet routinely and have decreased sensation as well as decreased peripheral circulation. One preventive measure is to have a husband and wife look at each other's feet, especially between the toes, searching for areas of infection or other suspicious findings. Prevention is an absolute necessity. The feet must be examined by both the diabetic patient and his physician. The "Ten Commandments of Foot Care" appear in the box below.

Damaged feet that previously would have been lost are now being saved because of better diabetic care, the use of antibiotics, and improved surgical techniques. Blood vessels that are not functioning well can be replaced surgically by utilizing grafts of blood vessels from other parts of the body or synthetic fiber vessels. Better foot care is available through physicians, podiatrists, nurses and even family members who are taught to monitor the feet. The best treatment is prevention. The quotation, "For want of a nail, the shoe was lost; for want of a shoe, the horse was lost; for want of a horse, the rider was lost" applies to foot care. The physician should be consulted at the first sign of inflammation, infection, trauma or discoloration.

TEN COMMANDMENTS OF FOOT CARE

1. *Never apply heat of any kind to the feet.*
2. *Never soak the feet.* Soaking the feet often allows too much time for the patient's skin and underlying structures to come in contact with excessive heat. Also, the skin is often macerated, and the barrier it provides to infection is broken. The old adage about soaking the feet in hot epsom salts solution "as long as one can stand it" is a *terribly dangerous directive for all diabetics of all ages at all times.*

3. *Never cut your own toenails; only file them.* The nails should be trimmed so that they are straight across and filed diagonally at the corners. Older nails are often thicker and in such cases, it is best to see a podiatrist. People who tend to have U-shaped nails may develop ingrown toenail problems. Periodic podiatric care is the best investment against foot problems.

4. *Never wear ill-fitting shoes.* Patients' vanity and commercialism have often allowed the medical aspects of good fitting to go unemphasized.

5. *Never go barefooted.* More injuries occur in the home when people do not wear footgear, be it shoes, slippers or clogs.

6. *Never assume that sensation or circulation is normal in the feet.* Often a vague numbness is the only sensation that patients with severe neuropathy describe. A survey of this problem showed that the healing of painless ulcers of the feet required more than three weeks of complete bed rest in a hospital, with all the maximal care this implies. These ulcers are not innocent lesions, despite the fact that they give no signal of trouble.

7. *Never use strong or colored medicines on the feet.* Strong medicines burn. Colored medicines, like Mercurochrome, are often ineffective and cover up areas of new inflammation.

8. *Never develop calluses or corns.* In general, this requires an appreciation of your particular foot problems to properly fit shoes.

9. *Never perform bathroom surgery on your own feet.* About as common as the problems related to ill-fitted shoes or injuries occurring when patients go barefoot are the self-inflicted wounds that occur when patients cut corns or use sharp scissors to cut the nails.

10. *Never keep the feet too moist or too dry.* Overly moist feet promote skin infections like athlete's foot. Overly dry skin allows fissures and cracks to develop and allows infection to enter. Keep a balance between the powdering and the lubricating of the feet.

skin problems

The skin covers the package known as the body and if the body has problems, the skin is likely to share these also. Diabetics have the same skin problems as others, as well as some problems specific to diabetes. One of these is excessively dry skin caused by dehydration in poorly controlled diabetes. Sometimes tiny areas known as "shin spots" (dermopathy) appear on the front of the legs. These are quite harmless, although worrisome. The increased incidence of athlete's foot and the possibility of fungus infection have already been discussed. Fatty plaques called xanthoma, orange-yellow in color, sometimes appear around the eyes or on the shins or elbows; they are usually related to high blood levels of fat and can be treated.

Probably the most specific problem for diabetics is a relatively harmless but cosmetically disfiguring condition called necrobiosis lipoidica diabeticorum, in which the layers of fat immediately below the skin disappear, so that the skin becomes discolored and dimpled. It occurs more often in girls than in boys, generally during the teen years, and although it may be found in other areas, it most often occurs on the front of the legs between the knees and ankles. It appears first as a pink discoloration and later becomes shiny and tight, much like the skin of an apple. The discoloration may be pink or red. This is very disturbing, particularly to young girls. However, the condition is not dangerous; the lesions often improve although this may require many years. Healing generally starts in the center of the lesion and then gradually extends to the sides. The danger is that the area may break open to form an ulcer and become infected.

There is no specific treatment. Ointments are generally useless, although improvements following the use of cortisone ointments have been reported. Skin grafts are sometimes necessary. Cover-ups or other cosmetic devices are often used to hide these unsightly blemishes. The wearing of slacks or pantsuits is helpful for women. However, the important thing is to recognize the presence of this condition.

psychological problems

The psychological problems of the long-term diabetic, discussed in detail later, may be formidable. The early lack of acceptance and resentment at having a chronic disease is understandable. The stages on the way to acceptance are: (1) fear and dismay; (2) relief at not having something worse; (3) a look at the future; and finally (4) acceptance and better care. However, after people have had diabetes for long periods, the greater risk lies in their becoming indifferent or too casual. Diabetics need support and understanding, not pity. Fortunately, most patients eventually adjust well.

summary

The long-term complications of diabetes may be threatening. However, many of these are not as formidable as they once were, owing to improved treatment. Eye problems continue, but with the use of the new generation of lasers and with more sophisticated research, much is being learned and the eyesight of many diabetics is being helped. There is also hope for people with kidney conditions. Neuropathy remains something of a mystery. Fortunately, although disabling and painful, it eventually improves. Remarkable advances have been made in vascular surgery to improve circulation to the feet. Thus, while there is much to learn about long-standing complications, the improvements in treatment are remarkable. Perhaps this is best exemplified by the statement of Dr. Priscilla White of the Joslin Clinic: when asked whether she was discouraged about the problems of long-term diabetics, she answered that if one considers only an individual patient, one might be discouraged, but if one considers diabetics as a group, they live not only longer and better than they did 25 years ago, but even ten or five years ago. Progress is being made!

Diabetes in the Young

10

Young people were never meant to have diabetes. At an age when they are full of enthusiasm and vigor and hope, it doesn't seem right for them to have a condition usually associated with older people. Children and young people are brave and accept acute illness with as much cheerfulness as possible, but they are not prepared to cope with something that appears to last forever. Very often the parents of the diabetic child are even less accepting about it. They may rise to the challenge of an acute disease or an accident, but the intrusion of something from another generation for which there currently is no cure appears to be the ultimate disaster. Moreover, nearly all parents of juvenile-onset diabetics appear to be totally overwhelmed at first. They often describe themselves as having been in a "state of shock" on learning about the diabetes in their child. Others seem to go through various stages, including resentment, denial and other phases, before adapting to and accepting the situation.

The new evidence that the onset of diabetes may be related to infections, probably of viral origin, lessens the personal trauma associated with the inheritance of diabetes. Many of the chemical and pathologic changes that characterize diabetes in the early stages of childhood can be produced by certain viruses in experimental animals. Present investigations are studying this relationship between viruses and onset in children. Diabetes today is not thought to be inherited simply as a Mendelian recessive trait coming through both sides of the family, but may be transmitted by many genes and many factors—it may be "multigenic and multifactoral."

Although increasing numbers of children are found to have diabetes, it is still, in this age group, relatively rare. Probably only about 4 to 5% of all diabetics are children, but the number increases as the total number of diabetics increases. The National Commission on Diabetes states that

600,000 new diabetics were diagnosed in 1974, and at the present rate the number of people with diabetes will double every 15 years. Although no one can accurately predict the future, all indications seem to imply that the numbers of youthful diabetics are increasing. The National Health Survey estimates the number of diagnosed diabetics under age 25 to be 1 in 1,000. Formerly the rate of diabetics under age 15 was reported to be one in 2,500 children. Analysis of the school records in Detroit, Michigan showed that one child in 500 was recorded as "diabetic." When those not requiring insulin were excluded, the rate was one in 650.

why do children develop diabetes

Assuming that infections superimposed on inheritance are important factors in the development of diabetes, other possible causes include the influence of anterior pituitary growth hormone, since significant numbers of youngsters become diabetic during their growth-spurts. At onset, diabetic children appear to be taller than their peers. The peak for onset of diabetes in girls is age 11 and for boys age 13, which suggests that the hormones related to puberty may be implicated.

In the Joslin Clinic series of more than 10,000 patients with known juvenile-onset diabetes, about one-third of the families knew of a relative with diabetes at the time of diagnosis, but after 20 years, 60% knew of such a relative, and after 40 years, about 75% of them knew of at least one relative with diabetes. Parents often deny the presence of any diabetes in the family, and indeed they may not know. This lack of real information about our forebears was treated deftly by Oliver Wendell Holmes (see box).

> Heredity is an omnibus in which all our ancestors ride, and every now and then one of them puts his head out and embarrasses us.
>
> —Oliver Wendell Holmes

In Dr. White's series, more cases of diabetes were diagnosed in January and July than in other months, possibly because during these months upper respiratory and gastrointestinal infections are more likely to enter and unmask the diabetes, or possibly affect the pancreatic islets in predisposed individuals.

The effect of heredity in juvenile diabetics is difficult to estimate. In the Oxford study (1946–47), several isolated juvenile diabetics were found. Fifteen years later, three generations of diabetes had been uncovered in each family, namely, the child, one of the parents and a grandparent.

natural history of diabetes in youth

Childhood diabetes is the classic form of diabetes and not surprisingly the signs and symptoms are very definite and often appear abruptly. At onset, these children have a tremendous thirst and sometimes urinate frequently both day and night. Bed-wetting may be an early sign of diabetes. The youngster's appetite is great, but in spite of drinking huge amounts of fluid and eating great amounts of food, he is never filled and often loses weight. (Later this ravenous appetite is lost.) These children are like a person suffering from thirst on a raft in the middle of a large body of water. They lose so much urine that they become dehydrated. Their vision blurs because of fluid loss from the eyeball. A formerly happy child becomes irritable and may unexpectedly do poorly in school. These children tire easily and sometimes have leg and abdominal pains. In contrast to adult-onset diabetics, who may knowingly have had diabetes for some time, the onset in children is most often sudden and dramatic, and the diagnosis is usually made shortly after the onset of symptoms, when greatly elevated blood sugar values of 300 to 500 mg. per cent are not uncommon. This is accompanied by large amounts of sugar in the urine. The fear of finding any glucose in the urine so impresses parents that they sometimes overread urine tests in the other children, not realizing that many nondiabetic children spill small amounts of glucose in urine without having diabetes. The diagnosis of diabetes in children is the same as for adults, although most often the onset is more dramatic. A glucose tolerance test is rarely needed for diagnosis of juvenile-onset diabetes. Occasionally, a youngster may have an adult-onset type of diabetes and then the glucose tolerance test is done; the amount of glucose given by mouth is adjusted downward for the lesser body weight.

Four distinct stages occur in juvenile-onset diabetes:
1. The acute onset.
2. Apparently lessened diabetes with possible remission.
3. Diabetes again becomes more intense.
4. Total diabetes.

In Dr. Priscilla White's series, 95% of children who develop diabetes under 15 years of age have "total diabetes" by the end of their fifth year of diabetes. As time goes on, the pancreatic beta cells become less and less effective, decrease in number and do not regenerate. Diabetes is sometimes more difficult to treat during periods of active growth or during infection.

Stage 1. At the time of diagnosis, there is still some insulin in the blood and pancreas. While the blood sugar levels may be elevated after meals, they often return to normal during the night.

Stage 2. The diabetes seems to improve and the patient's own insulin protection increases almost to normal amounts. This "remission" is a variable stage, but should not raise false hope or be interpreted wrongly as a "cure." Later, hope turns to despair when, as it nearly always does, the diabetes situation becomes more severe. Sometimes during this "remission" period, the patients seem to be able to be treated with diet alone or by some of the blood-sugar-lowering tablets. This remission period occurs in about one-third of the children, usually within three months after the beginning of treatment, and can last from several weeks to a year or more. Early intensive treatment seems to encourage this remission period, which comes to a close with further growth, gain in weight, infection, puberty or merely the passage of time.

Stage 3. When the diabetes becomes intense once again, parents are often discouraged. Blood sugar levels go up and down in spite of attempts at regulation. Unfortunately the battle that must be taking place in the beta and other cells of the body nearly always ends in the same way. The beta cells are overcome and the patient now is entirely dependent on insulin from outside sources.

Stage 4.   Total diabetes is the end result. No insulin can be found in the blood or pancreas, and the use and storage of food depend on the balance between food intake and available injected insulin. Presently, it is believed that growth hormone is an important factor in the onset of diabetes at this time. These patients are dependent on insulin regardless of age and will develop acidosis if insulin is omitted.

A common question at this time is "Will my child always have to take insulin?" The answer is almost always "yes," not because insulin is habit-forming, but because the child needs to replace the insulin that is not being made by his pancreas. When people lack thyroid, adrenal or ovarian hormones, these substances are replaced with thyroid extract, cortisone or estrogen. Insulin replacement is even more vital, because without insulin, metabolism could not take place and the patient could not survive.

differences between adult- and juvenile-onset diabetes

There are many differences between the diabetes of the young as compared to that of adults. Both the onset and clinical course are dissimilar, even though the basic condition is the same. In fact, some doctors feel that it is an entirely different kind of diabetes. This is not necessarily true. The difference may lie in the basic and complete lack of insulin in a growing child as compared to the metabolism of a static adult whose life processes are gradually deteriorating. If diabetes in the older person is like a fire in a smoldering pile of wet leaves, in the juvenile it often acts more like a raging dry-forest fire. Childhood diabetes is likely to be aggressive and unstable; adult-onset diabetes is usually much more stable.

In the youngster, there is complete expression of diabetes, and when this type of diabetes is conquered, adult diabetes will be better understood. In the adult, the onset can be very insidious with the result that some adults may have diabetes for five years or longer without ever being aware of the fact. On the contrary, the youthful onset of diabetes often is sudden and dramatic. Occasionally, atypical diabetes occurs in children with no obvious symptoms, and the diagnosis is based on blood sugar elevation during a glucose tolerance test just as in an adult. The fasting blood sugars may be normal. This might be an early stage of more severe diabetes and these patients have to be closely observed, although some have lived for many years without becoming overt diabetics. One example is a girl who had significant sugar in the urine at age 4 after scarlet fever. Over a period of 20 years, she never required more than 4 units of insulin. The insulin was later discontinued, but as she grew older the level of sugar in the urine increased and she required insulin during major surgery. She has elevated blood glucose levels during stress only. Sometimes diabetes in youngsters is as stable as that in many adults. However, these are rare exceptions. Furthermore, to prove that nothing is ever 100% certain in medicine, there are many adults who even at an older age have unstable juvenile-type diabetes.

treatment

While many grown-ups can survive with diet regulation alone, the typical juvenile cannot do so without insulin, whatever the diet. Admittedly, diet is still important in providing a foundation for satisfactory control, but insulin is absolutely life-saving.

Insulin.   In the young, even the use of insulin may be beset with problems. Theoretically, an intermediate insulin, such as Lente or NPH, should last 24 hours, but in children, more often than not, its action does not start soon enough nor does it last long enough. Therefore, in youngsters it is often necessary to combine the intermediate insulin with a fast-acting insulin, such as regular crystalline. Very early in diabetes, the intermediate insulin alone may regulate the condition. During the remission period, the insulin requirement may be very little, so that parents are tempted to eliminate it completely. However, it must never be eliminated, even if only 2 or 4 units daily are needed, for the following reasons. (1) Certainly, when the remission ends, insulin will be required, and it is simpler to increase the dose of insulin than to restart it. (2) False hopes should not be raised in the child about discontinuing insulin forever. (3) Although rare, discontinuing the injections of insulin, which is a protein, may sensitize the patient, so that in the future, resumption of insulin injections may cause an allergic-like response. A common problem for parents who are lulled by false hopes regarding the remission period is that they do not resume the injection of adequate doses of insulin even though the urine tests show increasing amounts of glucose.

In treating juveniles, a second dose of intermediate (NPH or Lente) insulin at bedtime is frequently necessary. While this may upset the child, it more often disturbs the parents, who believe that the diabetes is worsening. This is not true. The diabetes is starting to act the way it usually does. If the morning dose of intermediate insulin is increased too much in an attempt to continue its activity until the following morning, the child will almost certainly have severe hypoglycemic reactions during the peak of insulin activity, mostly in the late afternoon or evenings. The solution is to give a smaller amount of morning intermediate insulin and a second, still smaller injection at supper or bedtime. Often children need a combination of fast- and intermediate-acting insulins both before breakfast and before the evening meal. The other insulins, such as Semilente or Ultralente, may be used at the discretion of the physician. In juveniles, the very long-acting types of insulin such as protamine zinc, have not been satisfactory because of the possibility of severe insulin reactions occurring during sleep hours, which are always frightening.

Each child is an individual whose insulin program must be individualized. Parents sometimes become upset if their child takes more insulin than other youngsters. However, 40 units of insulin daily, for example, does not indicate that the diabetes is twice as severe as in someone taking 20 units. In fact, failure to increase the amount of insulin used daily as the child gets older may impair growth. On the other hand, insulin dosage that is excessive for a child's needs may predispose the child to such problems as low-blood-glucose reactions or obesity in adolescence.

None of the oral agents is effective in children.

Diet.   The days of severely limited diets for diabetic children are gone. The general principles are the same as for children without diabetes. The diet is planned to promote a normal rate of growth with enough calories for energy needs. A rough rule of thumb is approximately 1100 calories at age one, with 100 calories added each year up to the age of 19 for boys and 15 for girls. Many children need several diets: one for inactive days (such as school days), another with a 25% increase in calories for outdoor-exercise days, and another with a 25% decrease from the baseline diet for extreme inactivity or days of illness (see Sick Day Rules, Appendix 7).

The "free diet," which theoretically permits children to eat anything they wish, sounds attractive, but unfortunately it doesn't work for most juvenile diabetics. The balance between insulin, exercise and diet is a precarious one at best, and while some adults appear to thrive reasonably well in spite of an apparently careless diet, youngsters appear to have a much narrower tolerance, so that the diet or the meal plan becomes an important factor in maintaining reasonable diabetes regulation. Often, with a completely "free" diet on demand, the symptoms of diabetes recur. This can result in fatigue and weight loss. The diet for the growing child must be thoroughly adequate in protein, vitamins, minerals and calories. It is difficult to maintain any kind of management with a completely "normal" or "free" diet when one considers that an ordinary 17-year old boy could easily eat three-quarters of a loaf of bread heavily daubed with jam and butter.

A well-balanced, nondiabetic diet in the United States is usually a combination of 50% of the calories as carbohydrate, 15% as protein and 35% as fat. The traditional "diabetes" diet provides about 40% of the calories as fat, 20% as protein, and 40% as carbohydrate. Actually, either formula may be used as the basis for meal planning to achieve a consistent food intake, both through the day and also from day to day. The 50% carbohydrate figure is approximately that recommended by the American Diabetes Association Committee on Diet. The difference between the two diets is not so great, because it would actually amount to one more slice of bread or a medium fruit at each of the three meals daily. Admittedly, any upwards revision, especially in carbohydrate, adds to the difficulties in regulation. Remember that the goal of meal-planning is not to starve or deprive a child of food, but to provide all the food that is needed and that can be utilized by the body.

The food intake should be spread throughout the day, with about one-fifth of the calories taken at breakfast, two-fifths at lunch and two-fifths at the evening meal. Food for afternoon and bedtime snacks are either written into the meal plan specifically or subtracted from the noon and evening meals respectively. The purpose of the diet is to provide a stable intake with nearly the same amount each day, to provide sufficient nutrition during the active hours, and to avoid insulin reactions. The in-between-meal snacks should be adequate for active children. Modern foods are packaged reasonably accurately, and it is now easier to estimate amounts of food. It is amazing how adept a child becomes at measuring or estimating diet accurately. Once the onus of diabetes has been overcome and the condition accepted, children are often more at ease with diet therapy than their parents.

For weight-conscious adolescents, skimmed or "99% fat-free" milk is usable. Otherwise, normal foods are encouraged. Eggs are not as limited in growth diets during childhood as they might be in adults, but amounts of foods high in cholesterol are being reduced even in children. The tendency for diets in all youngsters, both diabetic and nondiabetic, is to greatly lower the fat content. It has been established that the obese adult has often started the process of obesity in childhood for many reasons: emotional, dietary or even ethnic or familial eating patterns, as described earlier. The more concentrated carbohydrate foods are limited. The aim is to try to keep the loss of sugar in the urine to less than 10% of the total carbohydrate intake for the day.

Exercise.   Most adults need motivation for regular exercise, but this is usually no problem with children. Exercise is actually a part of treatment. Activity after meals and quiet or rest periods before meals helps not only to control the peaks of blood and urine sugar levels, but also to avoid reactions. Neither the type nor the amount of exercise is restricted, but it is important to have snacks to prevent insulin reactions, especially when extreme activities such as swimming, ice skating or skiing are planned. Exercise also uses up blood sugar and can decrease the amount of insulin needed. This desirability for more exercise is one part of the treatment of diabetes that children never object to.

Understanding.   No one, whether adult or child, can be optimally treated for diabetes without love and understanding. With very young children, the parents must be educated concerning diabetes. The child and the parents must learn to respect but not be fearful of the condition. Other members of the family and friends as well must understand that the youngster with regulated or "controlled" diabetes is in good health. It is the preventable deviations from this state that cause difficulties and must be guarded against.

efforts at controlling diabetes

Unquestionably, the "control" of juvenile-onset diabetes is difficult. The belief that careful regulation of diabetes is not necessary arises from the fact that in many youngsters control is very difficult and almost impossible to achieve, especially if one considers that normal blood and urine glucose levels are the attempted ideal. In some patients who are not well versed in or may not accept the fundamentals of diet, mixed insulin and possibly split insulin doses, regulation can fluctuate so greatly that physicians may be tempted to look the other way as long as the patient "feels well." The problem is that much more is at stake besides "feeling well." The child's growth and development depend on the proper metabolism of food, as was obvious in the pre-insulin days. Even now with insulin injections available, improperly treated youngsters occasionally have enlarged livers that are filled with fat instead of stored glycogen. In the long-range view, those who have made an effort to maintain good regulation are found more frequently among the healthier long-term survivors who have lived 40, 50 or more years without severe complications.

Is it possible to keep the level of glucose in the blood normal throughout the 24 hours? Can the urine be kept free from sugar? In Stages 1 and 2, these objectives are possible. In Stage 3, an attempt is made to try to maintain ideal levels of blood sugar when fasting and before meals, and to try to limit the total amount of glucose lost in the 24-hour urine specimen to no more than 5% of the carbohydrate intake. In Stage 4 (total diabetes), the same goals are attempted, except that the amount of glucose lost in the urine is held to no more than 10% of the total sugar or starch intake in 24 hours. For example, if the diet provides 200 grams of carbohydrate daily, then 20 grams of sugar lost in 24 hours is acceptable. Of course, an attempt is made to avoid insulin reactions. In this way, the young person will have the energy and strength to continue his normal activities and grow normally.

Testing Urine Sugar.   Urine tests are an aspect of treatment that the child and the parents should understand. The significance of urine tests for children is the same as that for adults, except that juveniles often lose glucose in the urine in spite of normal blood sugar values. This may be due to a lowered "renal threshold," as discussed earlier. It sometimes also reflects rapid changes that occur in the blood glucose level, with a lag time before these changes become apparent in the urine tests. The best pattern of tests that a particular child can achieve needs to be determined by that child's physician, after a long period of observation. With current methods of treatment, almost no child with total diabetes has consistently normal blood glucose values.

The 24-hour urine test is important for youngsters. While it may not have to be performed frequently, it is the best measurement of what is happening to the level of sugar in the child's urine during a full 24 hours.

Testing Urine Acetone.   Urine acetone tests can be very important or very confusing. In nondiabetic children, acetone sometimes appears in the urine when, for example, a child has been playing vigorously in hot weather with not enough carbohydrate to be used as fuel, so the body uses some fat for this purpose. In diabetes, when large amounts of acetone appear along with significant amounts of sugar in the urine, it indicates a serious situation in which not enough insulin is available to use the glucose normally. Acetone under these circumstances becomes an indication of pending acidosis and possible disaster. Sometimes a small amount of acetone can be found in the urine during minor illness, with exercise or with insufficient food intake, and for other reasons. A good rule of thumb is to test for acetone only when the urine tests contain considerable amounts of glucose.

Testing Blood Sugar.   Although either a *venous* blood specimen (usually taken from the arm veins) or a *capillary* specimen (from the ear lobe or finger tip) may be used for testing blood sugar levels in children, the vein test is usually more accurate, even though it may be more difficult to obtain blood from the tiny veins of small children. However, the capillary blood test is accurate enough when performed in experienced laboratories, and it is much easier to obtain and causes less emotional upset. It is important to remember that one to two hours after a meal, the capillary blood (from the arterial supply) has glucose values that are 20 to 30 mg. per cent higher than the venous blood, because arterial blood contains glucose on its way *to* the cells while venous blood is returning *from* the cells, with much of the sugar already used. How often a child should have a blood sugar test depends on how well the physician or the parents can interpret the urine sugar tests. Some children have blood sugar tests performed once a month, and some less often. The "do-it-yourself" blood sugar test, Dextrostix (page 131), can be used to approximate the blood sugar level by using a color chart. It may be helpful during illness, while traveling or while at school or college.

what parents should know about diabetes

The parents of a new diabetic are frequently overwhelmed because, in addition to the understandable sorrow and occasional resentment at their child's diabetes, they may be thoroughly confused. The fancied intricacies of diet overwhelm them; the prospect of insulin reactions frightens them and, if the child is small, they are terrified at the thought of giving insulin. Most parents of new diabetics make the mistake of trying to learn at once everything there is to know about diabetes. This is neither possible nor necessary at the beginning of what is likely to be a life-long situation.

The parents should learn what the general plan and goals of treatment are and what has to be done to achieve them. Some of the more important early subjects are: (1) the technique of insulin injection and simple dose adjusting; (2) prevention and treatment of insulin reactions; (3) urine testing and its relationship to the insulin dose; (4) fundamentals of diet and how to provide the proper balance interestingly; (5) how to handle the child's diabetes during the generally short but frantic illnesses that come with childhood. This is not the time to worry about the possible foot problems of adulthood, eye problems, neuritis and other complications that may be related to long-term diabetes. Early, it is more important to encourage the participation of the child in diet and insulin therapy. For example, if there is no acute illness, insulin dose changes should be made when there is a trend in the urine tests for several days, rather than according to the findings each day. If the child understands the purpose of testing, there will be less misreporting of the results.

what the child must know

This depends on the age of the child, but most children can learn to inject their own insulin at almost any age. However, accurate regulation of the dose is a serious decision, which many children are not capable of making alone. It is probably not wise to let children assume complete responsibility for insulin dosage until at least age 12.

The child must understand the reasons for urine testing and should recognize the symptoms of the onset of a low-blood-sugar reaction and how to treat it. The child should also know the general goals and purposes of good treatment, so that he or she will be motivated to do what is best for himself or herself, rather than simply to please someone else.

emotional responses to diabetes

There are as many different responses to the onset of diabetes as there are people. In general, adults, once having accepted the diagnosis of diabetes, frequently take a philosophic attitude with grateful hearts that their condition is not a more threatening one. The attitude of children toward diabetes depends somewhat on the age group. Children under the age of five understandably protest the injection of insulin, although eventually they accept it, especially when they see others getting injections. Up through age 10, there is the problem of children relating to brothers and sisters who are not diabetic. The early teen-age years are periods of experimentation, often filled with emotional problems. Dr. Priscilla White points out that the initial stage is one of acceptance with a hope for complete cure or disappearance of the diabetes. When this does not happen, experimentation usually follows, then a period of denial of having diabetes, and eventually resignation or acceptance. To the despair of parents and others emotionally involved with these youngsters, the road from the first to the last-mentioned stage seems a long and tortuous one.

Behavior problems are discussed later (p. 211), but, in general, few young people are philosophically or emotionally prepared to accept diabetes as a lifetime pursuit without loving care and understanding from their parents and physicians.

complications

All of these complications have been previously discussed in Chapter 8; they are reviewed briefly here for the benefit of the young person with diabetes or the concerned family members.

Hypoglycemia (Insulin Reaction). The complications of diabetes early in its course are much the same in children as in adults, except that they can strike with such suddenness that they can be very frightening. Many of the commonest problems are those involving insulin therapy itself.

Insulin reactions (hypoglycemia) occur when the blood sugar level drops below normal and the symptoms are much the same as those discussed earlier, except for youth-adult differences. The child who is energetic may become quieter, while the quiet child often becomes agitated and unreasonable. Sometimes a child may become drowsy and with very low blood sugar levels, he may become unconscious. The skin may be sweaty, and since children develop convulsions easily, it is not uncommon to have convulsive-like seizures as a result of a sudden drop in blood glucose. While mild reactions are scarcely noticeable, violent reactions are frightening and the threat of these may cause apprehensive parents sleepless nights. Most insulin reactions are not dangerous. It is well to remember that anything that lowers blood glucose levels can cause symptoms of hypoglycemia, although in nondiabetics these are often overlooked. The irritability of the hungry adult and child alike may be related to low blood glucose. The child who eats too little lunch at school and plays hard on the way home becomes irritable or weepy about four o'clock in the afternoon. Mothers have learned that cookies and milk at this time are a wonderful antidote. Thus, while temporary personality changes due to a drop in the level of blood glucose may occur in both children and adults, these changes may be more sudden and much more definite in insulin-users.

Sometimes, in severe reactions, the convulsive seizures are

mistaken for those of epilepsy. Even brain wave tracings may show some changes. While some children do show epileptic tendencies, in most cases there is simply a lowered threshold for convulsions, which are triggered by low blood sugar levels. In a few cases the physician may prescribe mild sedative medications. Another symptom of insulin reaction, which is more typical of children than adults, is a gastrointestinal upset, which may result in vomiting.

The treatment of insulin reactions is the same for children as for adults. Six to eight ounces of orange or other fruit juice, ginger ale or a cola drink is helpful. In fact, honey, jelly or anything sweet and available can be used. If the child does not respond, the parents may inject a 1-cc. syringeful (1 mg.) of glucagon under the skin, just as with insulin. Half an ampule for a small child and up to two ampules (2 mg.) for a larger individual is the usual dose. Children also tolerate 0.1 to 0.3 cc. of 1:1000 solution of epinephrine (adrenaline) well in these emergencies. Severer forms of insulin reaction require the intravenous infusion of glucose by a physician. (See page 150.)

Ketoacidosis. This results with very high blood sugar levels, and is just the opposite of the insulin reactions described above. This complication has been described previously (see p. 157) and it is the same in children as in adults, except that in youngsters it occurs much, much faster, although never as rapidly as insulin reactions. A safe rule of thumb is that if disorientation or unconsciousness develops very suddenly, it is more likely due to an insulin reaction.

Although childhood ketoacidosis has occurred in only 10% of Joslin Clinic patients, 40% of the patients admitted to the New England Deaconess Hospital in ketoacidosis or coma have juvenile-onset diabetes. Modern treatment methods have reduced the percentage of deaths due to coma from over 60% to about 1%. This is the most perilous acute complication of diabetes.

Insulin Abscesses and Infections. These can develop because of careless injection technique. They may be small and may be treatable with antibiotics, or they can develop into quite large areas that may require surgical treatment. They are always preventable.

Fat Atrophy. Disappearance of fat tissue just under the skin at or near the sites of insulin injection is very upsetting to the child, and even more upsetting to the parents who think this will happen all over the body. Actually, it doesn't; this is self-limited and such areas will improve in 99% of children, although it may take years. It occurs less frequently with the newer and purer insulins.

Fat Hypertrophy. Tissue sometimes builds up in the areas of insulin injection, usually on the thighs. This is called hypertrophy, and it is just the opposite effect of atrophy. It is a harmless complication.

Insulin Allergy. This condition resembles hives with local itching and swelling as well as redness. It is caused by insulin allergy and is not uncommon in children early in diabetes treatment.

Insulin Edema. Occasionally young persons under treatment with insulin develop swelling around the ankles. This is caused by the accumulation of fluid in the body. It is rarely severe, although it may frighten the new diabetic. Sometimes the physician may prescribe diuretic drugs temporarily to remove the fluid.

Some of the other problems are much like those that occur in adults. Local infections as a result of poor technique and hygiene, of course, are possible at any age. Response to the appropriate treatment is good.

The long-duration diabetic may be susceptible to changes in the tiny blood vessels of the eyes and kidneys. These do not frequently occur under age 20 or before 12 to 15 years of diabetes. These are discussed in Chapter 9.

Newer developments offer hope for minimizing or treating these problems. It is the diabetic children of the world who have made the most obvious progress towards a happy life. The wan, scrawny, hungry youngster, such as those portrayed by Charles Dickens, no longer describes the child with diabetes, thanks to modern care. Furthermore, with adequate diets and more modern eating plans, the plaintive, "Please sir, may I have some more?" of Oliver Twist days is not necessary for the young with diabetes.

growth and development

Diabetics are often superior children. They are healthy, intelligent and attractive. The records of Dr. Priscilla White, collected over many decades, show that youngsters who develop diabetes often have excellent growth and health. Today parents and children can be reassured that growth and development will progress in normal fashion. Between the years 1922 to 1940, one boy in four with diabetes and one girl in ten showed failure in growth, as much as 4 to 13 inches below the standard average for the age. Such children were known as "diabetic dwarfs" and these were most often those whose diabetes began at age five to ten years or earlier. Such children had, in addition to growth failure, very large fat-infiltrated livers, sometimes causing abdominal pain. X-ray pictures of the leg bones showed the presence of many horizontal lines when growth did not take place. The onset of puberty was also delayed. These children were intelligent and did well in school.

The development of the long-acting insulins has improved growth and development by providing many more hours of control of the metabolism of carbohydrate, protein and fat. This could also have been accomplished if regular insulin had been used, but because of its shorter duration of action, four or more injections of insulin would have been required daily. Even today, if insufficient insulin is used, one child in 100 shows this tendency to diabetic dwarfism. With better treatment, the enlargement of the liver is reduced and growth progresses as it should. All boys are concerned about height and diabetic boys are no exception. Of course, some people are shorter than others with or without diabetes, and for this trait, our ancestors should be blamed, particularly in these days of better nutrition when children in general are taller than they used to be. However, growth and development are no longer diabetic problems provided an adequate diet is furnished and good control of diabetes maintained.

Diabetic Babies.   Babies with diabetes are very rare, but increasingly diabetes is being found in younger age groups. A diabetic baby can compound problems. Mothers become very adept at testing the baby's urine by wringing out diapers or using TesTape on the diaper. The very young survive well with amazingly small amounts of insulin, as low as 2 to 4 units daily. These children will always need insulin, in increasing amounts, as they grow and develop.

Puberty. In those who develop diabetes at an early age, the development of puberty may be delayed. This causes anxiety and distress among parents. Normal development of puberty in a girl consists of the rounding of the hips, more specific breast development, the appearance of pubic and axillary hair, and finally the beginning of the menstrual cycle. The delayed onset of menstruation and long periods without menses upset both the girls and their mothers. Those who develop diabetes after age 11 may have an early onset of menstrual periods. Of course, irregular cycles are not uncommon in all girls up to age 17, even in those without diabetes. By age 19, if irregularities persist, a cause other than diabetes should be considered and investigated by the physician. A common reason for delayed menstrual periods is a lack of thyroid hormone (hypothyroidism). Families should realize that delay of regular menstrual cycles is not harmful. Eventually the periods do occur, and certainly diabetic women have normal sex lives and are able to conceive and bear children like anyone else.

In boys, the development of puberty consists of the growth of the testes, enlargement of the penis, the growth of pubic, axillary and body hair, and deepening of the voice. This onset is also variable with nondiabetics as well.

Effect of Menstrual Periods. During menstruation the kidney threshold for losing glucose in the urine may be reduced, causing confusion with regulation of diabetes. A patient may complain of having insulin reactions and yet have glucose in the urine. Acidosis is not brought on by menstruation; if it does occur, reasons other than the menstrual period have caused it. There is no doubt, however, that menstrual periods can make diabetes control a bit more difficult for a few days each month.

school

All children, including diabetics, certainly must attend school. While it is important for the growing child to have as good diabetes regulation as possible, it is also important to maintain blood glucose levels high enough to prevent insulin reactions during active periods such as traveling to school, recess, sports and other periods of sometimes frenetic activity.

The teacher should be aware of the diabetes, but should not shelter or overly protect the youngster. Most of all, teachers must not make obvious special allowances for the diabetes. Children do not want to appear different from their classmates. Occasionally psychologically traumatic episodes occur, as, for example when a child is hospitalized and the well-intended but poorly informed teacher announces to the class, "Johnny is diabetic. We must watch him very carefully and help any way we can. If he does something strange, please let me know right away." Certainly this child would be disturbed by unwanted attention when he returns to school.

What is told the schoolteacher is most important to the child and his diabetes. There should be enough information, but not too much. Mostly the fact of diabetes, the possibility of insulin reactions and their treatment are important. It is also important that the teacher permit snack-times as necessary without fanfare. The needed information can be printed on cards for distribution to the school teachers. One type in use is shown in Figure 31.

parents' groups

It would not be fair to stress the psychologic effect of diabetes on the psyche of the young without mentioning the problems of their parents. Their adjustment is often as stormy or stormier than that of their youngster with diabetes. In addition to the fears and problems of caring for their child, they may harbor a sense of guilt that becomes manifest in many directions. Recently groups of parents have been meeting not only for ventilation of their problems, but for mutual consideration of means of coping. When they have proper guidance by trained persons who are capable of helping their psychological as well as emotional needs, the results have been gratifying.

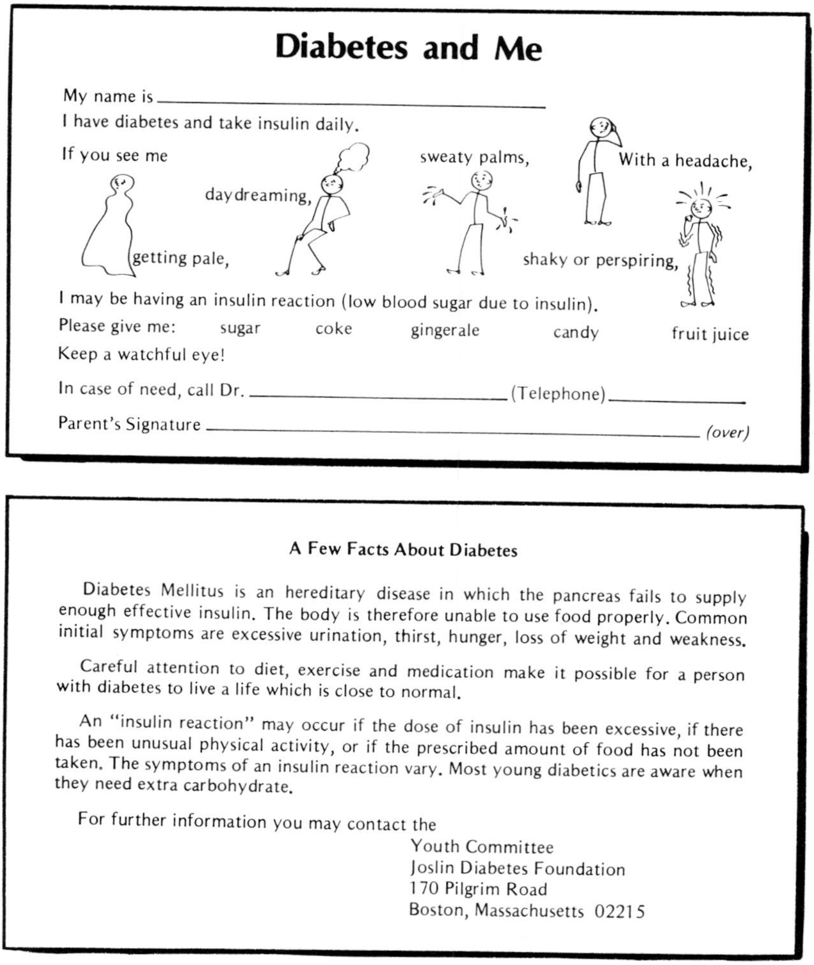

Diabetes and Me

My name is _____

I have diabetes and take insulin daily.

If you see me   daydreaming,   sweaty palms,   With a headache,

getting pale,   shaky or perspiring,

I may be having an insulin reaction (low blood sugar due to insulin).

Please give me: sugar   coke   gingerale   candy   fruit juice

Keep a watchful eye!

In case of need, call Dr. _____ (Telephone) _____

Parent's Signature _____ (over)

A Few Facts About Diabetes

Diabetes Mellitus is an hereditary disease in which the pancreas fails to supply enough effective insulin. The body is therefore unable to use food properly. Common initial symptoms are excessive urination, thirst, hunger, loss of weight and weakness.

Careful attention to diet, exercise and medication make it possible for a person with diabetes to live a life which is close to normal.

An "insulin reaction" may occur if the dose of insulin has been excessive, if there has been unusual physical activity, or if the prescribed amount of food has not been taken. The symptoms of an insulin reaction vary. Most young diabetics are aware when they need extra carbohydrate.

For further information you may contact the
Youth Committee
Joslin Diabetes Foundation
170 Pilgrim Road
Boston, Massachusetts 02215

FIG. 31. This simple card, designed by the Youth Committee of Joslin Diabetes Foundation, is one useful type of information to be carried by the primary grade school student.

parties

Parties are major events in the lives of all children. As mentioned earlier, the diabetic child must not be stigmatized as being "different," and the poorest possible approach is to have the hostess in anyway make an issue of the diabetes. The daily diet can be adjusted to permit ice cream or some plain cake on this special occasion. If necessary, some supplemental insulin could be used before or after the party. Unless one makes a career of partying, the resentment engendered in the young person is probably more harmful to the diabetic career than the temporary allowed-for alterations in "control" on unusual occasions. It is far better for the youngster to adjust to the circumstances than to suffer a blow to the ego. Common sense on the part of the parents and understanding by the child are better than an impossibly rigid set of conditions.

travel

In this jet age, travel is an important part of the life of many families. Whether this means an educational trip overseas, a camping trip or any other prolonged stay away from home, there is no reason why young diabetics should not have a normal life style in this regard. This is discussed extensively in the travel section in Chapter 11 (page 246). The young, with or without diabetes, can travel almost anywhere and be able to participate in overnight hikes, camping and skiing as well as other activities of youth. Parents often fear the insulin reactions and the other possible difficulties that their children with diabetes might have to endure. For the child, diabetes is almost always a lifetime matter that will have to be fitted into his or her lifestyle at home and outside the home.

Of course, the reverse problem can be distressing when the parents are fearful of going away from home and abandoning their "sick" child. Time is well-spent in teaching a trustworthy babysitter, nurse or whoever is in charge of the children to recognize and treat insulin reactions. The phone number of the family physician as well as the location of the parents should be left in an obvious place. There is no great problem with older children in this respect, but even with the very young, it is important not to have the parents' fears change the course of what should be a normal, happy life for the whole family.

camps and youth centers

Camps and youth centers are used primarily for vacations and for changes in routine. These may be either regular camps with special facilities or ability to supervise and care for diabetics, or camps primarily devoted to children with diabetes. Such camps are the Elliott P. Joslin Camp for boys at Charlton, Mass., and the Clara Barton Birthplace Camp for girls three miles away in North Oxford, Mass. in the rolling green country 50 miles west of Boston. Older teenagers and young adults are employed as counsellors, program directors and other staff members. Some believe that the diabetes camp program is not good because it isolates the diabetic child among his own kind. These persons believe that it is better for a diabetic to learn to take care of himself among nondiabetic children. This may be true for the secure, well-indoctrinated and self-assured older diabetic, but a much greater feeling of security as well as camaraderie exists among diabetic children who play together, work together and, more importantly, learn together. Camp relieves the anxiety and depression that many children experience about being different and good diabetic treatment can be carried out under ideal conditions of exercise and activity. With teaching by counsellors, nurses and the camp physician, the child returns home not only healthier, but better informed and prepared for life. Such camps provide many children with their first opportunity to learn about their diabetes and also have the added dividend of providing their parents with several carefree weeks away from their children, knowing that they can safely forget their responsibilities for a time. Many diabetes camps have now been established in the United States, Canada and Europe.

sports and activities

Sports, both organized and casual, are encouraged for diabetics. The coach of a team and the teammates should know of the possibility of insulin reactions, but with simple precautions and increased food on days of heavy activity, diabetics should, within their own abilities, take part in nearly every type of sport. These activities are not only beneficial mentally, but help to use extra blood glucose, often necessitating smaller doses of insulin. Diabetics can ski, swim, play tennis and engage in most activities, although certain sports such as swimming or scuba-diving, during which an insulin reaction could prove dangerous, should always be done in the company of others who know about the diabetes. It is imperative that the diabetic use the "buddy system" during such activities.

"growing pains;" behavioral problems

A quick look at contemporary life makes it plain that teenagers and developing people, like developing countries, may have very special problems. Teenagers, buffeted as they are by the changes that occur in the transition from puberty to adulthood, may have emotional problems. It should not be surprising that the addition of a chronic condition that requires continued painstaking care does little to make life smoother for this group. Behavior problems, as already pointed out, begin in the youngest diabetics, and while they vary with different age levels, they may become more profound in adolescents. The normal anxieties of adolescence are amplified by the realities of life. The teenager must understand about insulin, reactions, testing, diet and precautions that the ordinary young person would either rather forget about or have someone else take care of for him.

Falsification of Tests.   The very young can accept the rules laid down by their parents. Falsification of tests by an older child in an attempt to win the parents' approval or to keep them from nagging him can lead to disaster. It is important not to overemphasize or make a fetish of "blue tests," since some children, reaching for approval, will simply carry out their tests using tap water or conveniently misreport the results. (This practice is not limited to youngsters.) Parents cannot understand why the urine glucose tests are constantly sugar-free at home, while in the physician's office both the urine and blood glucose levels are greatly elevated.

At a later age, the insulin doses may be manipulated. Sometimes early teenagers secretly take extra insulin to have sugar-free urine tests continually in an attempt to please the physician and obtain the praise of their parents. They may deny taking extra insulin, and sometimes youngsters have been admitted into a hospital with a diagnosis of severe insulin reaction and a history of "no insulin given." These situations are eventually unraveled. The psychological reasons for these occurrences should be sought and treated. These episodes most often occur with girls, who are often more complex and inventive than boys of the same age. One girl indulged in an escapade of this type and confused the attending medical staff for nearly a week. When the hidden syringe, needles and insulin were discovered and the parents confronted, the mother's reaction was "Why would she do a thing like this to me?" This inappropriate response pinpointed the problem neatly. In this particular family, the diabetic child was jealous of an attractive sister who had many dates. She used the diabetes as a weapon to force the family to focus attention on her. These are not criminal acts, but the cries of young people who want understanding and compassion.

It is difficult for parents with their anxieties not to overindulge the diabetic child or, conversely, insist on a regimen that is too strict and unrealistic. Rarely is the diabetic child neglected; more often the tendency is toward overprotection. The solution to many of these problems is to work personally with the diabetic child and early teenager. Frequent discussions and small talk about the adjustments of insulin dosage will strengthen the understanding that the purpose of the tests is not to bring on praise or punishment, but to permit the proper amount of insulin. An important point for parents: blood or urine tests should not be referred to as "good" or "bad" tests. This is not a moral issue. The urine glucose tests have "no sugar" or are "positive for sugar" in varying degrees.

Teenagers should be responsible for their own insulin doses after consultation with the parents and physician but the rules must not be impossibly rigid. A single meaningful and accurate urine glucose test once daily, or several in one day, may be enough in the stabilized diabetic. The "teens" are not always geared for fastidious details of testing. Unquestionably, three or four urine tests for glucose are most desirable, but, it is better to have the patient's cooperation with fewer and more meaningful tests than to have no testing or careless testing. In time, the previously rejected idea of urine testing might be accepted.

Sibling Rivalry. Sibling rivalry, which may start early, can continue into later years. Strangely, the diabetic does not resent brothers and sisters nearly as much as the nondiabetics may resent the one with diabetes. This may be because it is difficult for parents not to give the diabetic extra attention, and youngsters in the family mistake the extra attention for favoritism.

Experimentation. Many early teenagers are experimenters and diabetics are no exception. This experimentation may involve diet and insulin as well as relationships with friends and parents. It is most important for the youngster to realize the importance of insulin and diet. A few days of neglecting insulin may convince the child of its importance.

Peer Approval. Most youngsters are peer-worshippers in the early teens. They seek the approval of their friends and do not want to be different. Whether the current fad is sloppy clothes or neat pinstripes, shaggy hair or crewcuts makes little difference, since the youngsters shun individualism. (Later in life, they may emerge as adults who drive sport cars, wear absurd hats, or brag about their surgical incisions at cocktail parties to bring attention to their "uniqueness.") Young people with chronic conditions other than diabetes have also been known to ignore the proper care for their disease, with disastrous results.

Denial. Early adolescence is also an age of denial for all young persons, including those with diabetes. However, around the ages of 17 to 20, young people begin to take a different attitude toward life in general and their own careers in particular, and start to think of college, employment and marriage, which may help them to overcome denial of their diabetes. In the meantime, they have driven their parents up the wall with anxiety!

Rejection. When denial is extreme, rejection of diabetes may take place. The patient denies that diabetes exists at all. This ability of young diabetics to delude themselves may even deceive their parents as well as their physician, since it may be difficult to detect this attitude. Parents, when confronted with the evidence, often refuse to accept the possibility of denial, falsification of tests or experimentation, because they think these behaviors reflect on them.

Parents and children must understand that, in the typical

diabetes of the young, it is not easy to have urine tests without sugar, especially as the islets of Langerhans cease insulin production. The parents must understand that the child is really trying, if indeed he is. Confidence begets confidence. Young people must have reasons for testing. At this age, anything foreign to the usual lifestyle (such as testing urine for sugar) can be odious. In contemporary language, it is not their "bag." Yet many children, whose parents believe they have no interest in their own care, may take more interest than is apparent.

Depression occurs in adolescents readily enough, and it is still more common in adolescents with diabetes. They are often aware of death and disability, and fear that their lives are going to be shortened by diabetes. They may feel that they may as well have a fling and live life to the full, disregarding all precautions. The more they learn about diabetes and are permitted to make decisions in their treatment, the better the results will be. As young diabetics realize that pretending that the condition does not exist accomplishes nothing, they often take much more interest in treatment and better care of themselves.

drinking, smoking, drugs

Sometimes the young person further complicates his life by drinking, smoking or taking drugs. These are discussed in Chapter 11.

education and employment

As the child with diabetes becomes an adult, he becomes concerned with further education, classical or vocational. Colleges don't exclude young people with diabetes, although some postgraduate schools have not encouraged enrollment of diabetic students, perhaps as a result of unrewarding experiences with other diabetics. Young diabetics have successfully attended colleges, postgraduate schools, technical training and business schools. Many states support these young people in full or in part, usually through a department of rehabilitation. Academic records have been good. The rehabilitation commissions are usually federally funded but administered by each state individually, sometimes under the education, mental health, or other departments. As with many state-administered federally-funded programs, there are great differences in the funding and administrative practices among states because the rules vary with each jurisdiction. In Massachusetts, for example, the title is Commonwealth of Massachusetts Rehabilitation Commission.

Increasingly, greater employment and new careers are open to diabetics, although certain positions in which hypoglycemic reactions might be harmful to the individual or others are obviously excluded. This topic is discussed further under "Career Guidance" (page 225). Some employers are reluctant to hire individuals with diabetes because of increased insurance costs that sometimes penalize those who hire anyone with chronic health conditions. This is unfortunate and unfair to those with diabetes who take good care of themselves and have dependable work records.

the youth committee

Because of the problems peculiar to diabetic young people, they are in a good position to understand each other's problems and to suggest acceptable solutions. For this reason a Youth Committee was formed at the Joslin Diabetes Foundation. This consists of young diabetics whose onset of diabetes started as children. They exchange ideas and information and discuss topics of mutual concern. A specially trained Youth Counselor is available to help organize and coordinate their activities.

marriage

Like nearly everyone else, most diabetics will marry. It is useful for diabetics considering marriage to have genetic counseling and certainly the prospective nondiabetic partner should be aware of the possible problems and complications. The prospective married couple should also be aware of the everyday emergencies that can take place. Husbands and wives of diabetics as well as those who plan to marry diabetics should attend classes for diabetes instruction, so they will be able to cope without fear.

A physician in Europe theorizes that those with diabetes should only marry one another because this would eventually limit diabetes to a smaller and smaller segment of the population and also because the husband and wife would understand each other's problems. It is very unlikely that this idea will ever become very popular. Rarely have two young people in love ever been dissuaded by reason or logic, and love being what it is, people will probably simply continue to marry whomever they choose. The least that can be done is to provide them with the best information and help possible. (Further discussion of marriage and childbearing appears in Chapter 11, page 240.)

why try to control diabetes in the young

Much has been learned in the understanding of diabetes, and long duration of life for those whose onset of diabetes occurred in childhood is common. Some patients with diabetes onset dating from before the discovery of insulin have lived longer than 50 years. One of these, a 70-year-old woman with 58 years of diabetes, is in excellent health. Another man is 60 years of age with a duration of 52 years of diabetes, and a third developed diabetes at the age of 4 and is now age 60. Many juvenile-onset diabetics in good general health have survived longer than 40 years in the Joslin Clinic series. Most of these have lived satisfactory, productive and unsheltered lives.

Many parents understandably are concerned and ask "How long will my child live?" They point to the longevity tables, which state that the "average diabetic" life duration is nearly 30 years. If their child started with diabetes at age 5, does this mean that the child will not live past the age of 35? This is not true. The statistics quoted refer to the average duration of life after onset of diabetes in those who have died; they do not take into account the many, many others who are living on and on. Furthermore, for everyone who lived less than 30 years, someone else lived longer than 30 years. This is how averages are derived. It is still too early in the insulin era

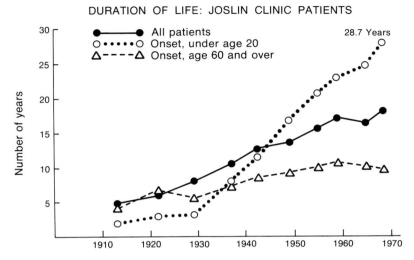

DURATION OF LIFE: JOSLIN CLINIC PATIENTS

●———● All patients
○•••••○ Onset, under age 20
△----△ Onset, age 60 and over

28.7 Years

FIG. 32. Since the discovery of insulin, diabetics of all age groups have had a remarkable increase in longevity, but the greatest increase occurs in those who became diabetic as juveniles. The rate of nearly 30 years of life is an average, based only on death rates from all causes. It does not include the number of living diabetics, and for each person who lived less than the average, another lived longer.

to determine the life expectancy of the diabetic child or adolescent who has had insulin available to control diabetes from its onset. (See *Fig. 32.*)

It is known that most diabetics can live a full and fruitful life. How *well* they live it depends on how much they know about their diabetes and how well they take care of themselves. While youngsters would rather be free of any responsibility or care, those who have taken the best possible care have survived best. The younger diabetic has much to look forward to, because in recent years, not only have treatment methods improved and diets become more generous, but many complications now can be treated successfully. Recent developments and research progress offer ever-increasing hope.

Living with Diabetes

11

There is only one purpose in good care for diabetics and one reason for learning everything possible about diabetes: to keep the diabetic in the best of health. However, the *quality* of life is as important as the *length* of life. Since the fact of diabetes will not simply disappear, it becomes important for the diabetic to live well with diabetes. It is difficult to really achieve a victory over any chronic condition until the fact of that condition is accepted.

acceptance

No diabetic person can live quite as normally as a nondiabetic person. Complete freedom to eat and be as active as one chooses at any time is restricted by a program that must follow the action of the daily insulin injection. Naturally, having to abide by this daily plan, which requires needles, syringes, a new or revised diet and a continued concern over infections, skin care and health in general, invokes strong emotional feelings. The individual's response is influenced, of course, by age and also by the nature of the onset of diabetes. Equally important are the help (or lack of it) offered by friends, family or physicians and the number of threatening medical situations that occur. However, a major clue to the happiness of the diabetic patient is his degree of acceptance of the disease. This acceptance depends on the ability of each individual patient to cope. The ways in which people adapt to diabetes must be understood if acceptance is to be gained.

Denial. This mechanism is a universal and natural response to an undesirable problem like diabetes. "Denial" usually is the main reason for neglect of good health advice by patients in general. Even normal people go through life intermittently denying all sorts of real situations. When diabetes occurs, the patient's denial may take several forms. Few people dare deny the existence of the condition totally by skipping or purposely confusing insulin doses. However, many people neglect their diabetes relatively by taking too little insulin, by making too few preventive visits to their physician and by living with a self-destructive behavior that displays chronic rather than acute neglect. Some social traditions make it easy for some people to deny their problem. Patients sometimes say, "I deny my diabetes all of the time except for 15 minutes in the morning when I take my insulin shot." As people mature, they learn to deny less, to face their problems and to follow the required treatment in a resigned but certainly not depressed fashion. Education is often helpful in resolving this problem. Ideally, patients will learn enough to say "Now I know that I can lead a better life by taking responsibility for my care and improving it." Group experiences with other diabetics, whether at camps for children with diabetes, counselling for young adults by "big brother" or "big sister" volunteers, or discussion groups for adult diabetics, can help break through patterns of denial.

Fear.   Information about diabetes often confuses patients. Some of the statistics about diabetes, or some examples of individual diabetics who fared poorly, may produce fear. Many families recall the experiences of past family members who had an unfortunate experience with their diabetes, even though the previous situation *may not* relate to the new diabetic person's situation. More often than not, these memories have an unfavorable and negative influence on the new patient's concept of his own condition. Anxiety is a natural result of this type of influence. Hope can be generated by good advice. The use of correct insulin dosages that really make the patient feel better and learning about diabetics who have successfully taken care of themselves will help to encourage the newly diagnosed diabetic. If such positive influences do not help, anxiety can become an all-consuming way of life for the diabetic and influence relationships with family, spouse and working partners. Furthermore, young people with diabetes often rebel when parents remain overanxious and therefore overprotective. Some people submit to this fear and anxiety and live a dull, defeated lifestyle that so bogs down their

thinking that they are incapable of making important decisions.

    Guilt. Guilt is the third most common response to the
diagnosis of diabetes. Certainly, if the hereditary aspects of
diabetes are truly understood, any acceptance of guilt by one
parent or transfer of guilt to the other parent makes no sense.
Still, patients and their families sometimes harbor beliefs that
through diabetes they are somehow suffering for previous
misdeeds or "sins." This primitive feeling makes people depressed and less able to handle the daily requirements of living
with diabetes. People should remove diabetes from the realm
of morals. Guilt is rarely a successful, long-term means of
motivation.

    If these feelings of denial, fear and guilt can be adequately
expressed and discussed, a better perspective of the situation
and acceptance may be achieved. Overcoming the natural
emotional feelings about having diabetes is a major concern of
doctors, nurses and those family members who are trying to
help their diabetic friends and relatives.

how long will I live

Statistics regarding the duration of life for the diabetic patient
are often either misquoted or misinterpreted, as well as mis-
understood. The way in which statistics are reported in newspapers and books often causes severe anxiety in readers. With
the proper use of insulin, antibiotics, and other modern drugs
when required, as well as earlier diagnoses and generally
better treatment, diabetics live longer than ever before, and
each new development creates hope for further extension of
life. Increasing numbers of diabetics are living 50 years or
more. Of course, persons who develop diabetes at advanced
ages are not going to survive 50 years no matter how meticulous their treatment, since even superb care won't guarantee
immortality, but most diabetics who survive for long periods
have juvenile-onset diabetes. Even more important, the life-
duration curve is still increasing, especially for juvenile-onset
diabetics. While it is still not correct to say that diabetics live
as long as nondiabetics overall, without question the statistics
have improved.

One factor that causes those with diabetes to become discouraged is the attitude that one can do little to influence the future. This is not true. A person with diabetes can make the future less favorable in at least three areas:

1. Delaying diagnosis and treatment.
2. Neglecting treatment or having inadequate treatment.
3. Neglecting other factors that influence illness states and may shorten life. For example, if a young diabetic also has a family history of high blood pressure, yet despite this fact he is overweight and smokes heavily, he may have a shorter lifespan than if he were an active person, weighed less and did not smoke.

Diabetes is not a predictable disease, but a mixture of abnormalities that express themselves at different rates in different persons. Such disorders are more difficult to evaluate and predict than individual conditions like infections. In considering the prospects for the future, one must not concentrate on the past experiences of individual diabetics, but consider instead the overall improvement of the group in general.

education of the diabetic

Education is not an addition to treatment, it *is* treatment. Without it, the patient is unable to handle the treatment tools that are his ultimate salvation. Understanding even the simplest diet or the injection of insulin requires knowledge. The lives of diabetics worldwide would be enormously better if every newly-discovered diabetic were taught to understand diabetes.

How much should a patient know? This depends on the person's understanding, ability and motivation. Basic facts regarding diet, insulin injection, treatment of reactions, avoidance of infection and acidosis, sick-day rules and foot care are the fundamentals that will enable the patient to survive. A new diabetic should not be overwhelmed by over-education with unnecessary information at the beginning. The long-term subtleties can be learned later.

How does the diabetic learn the facts? Primarily it is the responsibility of the physician and the teaching team to instruct the patient and his family. The team is made up of nurses, dietitians, and other health professionals, a group now identified as "diabetes educators." Hospitals and other institutions provide teaching as well as educational material. Another source of information is the American Diabetes Association publication, *Diabetes FORECAST,* available by subscription. Every diabetic should belong to an affiliate of the American Diabetes Association. These local groups have access to speakers and programs, and members learn from one another and help each other. Other groups, such as the Juvenile Diabetes Foundation, promote research to help younger diabetics. If such voluntary health organizations involved with diabetics could unite, they could exert a powerful force for good. The Joslin Diabetes Foundation also provides educational materials.

choosing a physician

Who should your doctor be? Probably 90% of diabetics have been and will continue to be treated by a personal physician, whether a family practitioner or an internist. It is important to have a physician who is experienced in diabetes and interested in the patient. The good general physician who is concerned about his patients and their needs knows when to refer them to specialists for help. If a physician particularly trained in diabetes is available, so much the better, but it is important to have a doctor who knows you, who cares, and who can and will spend time with you. Also, don't wait to see a physician until an emergency arises. Unfortunately, the chronic character of diabetes often lulls both patient and physician into a state in which minimal problems may be overlooked; these often become greater problems if neglected.

how often to see your physician

This depends on your physician. During periods of poor control or when adjustment is needed, visits may be weekly or monthly. Stable diabetics with sufficient knowledge to assume responsibility for much of their own care may need to be seen only a few times yearly. Most important is good record-keeping of urine tests. The more accurate the medical records available to the physician, the better will be the advice and care. Some physicians have patients mail them the results of a series of tests at intervals.

the economics of diabetes

Diabetes can be expensive. The diabetic diet, with its emphasis on protein rather than carbohydrate, may be somewhat costlier than a nondiabetic diet. Medical care can also be costly. Likewise, insulin and the necessary equipment for injection are an unceasing expense, as are oral hypoglycemic agents. Sometimes, because of job discrimination, diabetics may have diminished incomes. Some employers hesitate to hire diabetics because of (1) ignorance, (2) a previous bad experience with a diabetic employee or (3) insurance or retirement programs that may require increased premiums to cover persons with conditions like diabetes.

A national health survey recently disclosed that 37% of known diabetics were actively employed, 38% were women homemakers and 16% were retired. The rest (nearly 10%) fell into the category of "others," which included children and the unemployed and disabled. Later data showed that nearly 60% of male diabetics of age 17 and over were employed. Nevertheless, diabetics seeking employment sometimes have difficulties, even though recent data from employers such as Ford and Dupont show that diabetic employees have a remarkably good work record. Working diabetics also have the responsibility to improve their image as good workers. Dr. Paul S. Entmacher of the Metropolitan Life Insurance Company states that the diabetic job applicant should not conceal his diabetes under any circumstances and suggests that it is helpful to bring to the employment office a physician's report of diabetes control or, for younger people, a good school attendance report. The medical department of the place of employment should be aware of the diabetes and the medications used. The diabetic's co-workers should also be aware of the possibility of hypoglycemic reactions and how to treat them. Accidents may occur if a diabetic has an insulin reaction and fellow employees are not knowledgeable about it. The diabetic should initiate a "buddy" system to ensure that he receives prompt help when needed.

Career Guidance. Career guidance is important for diabetics. Certain jobs are understandably not open to diabetics. Recently, diabetics using insulin have been prohibited from driving large trucks in interstate commerce. Cities, towns and states sometimes have regulations regarding public transportation jobs, such as locomotive engineers or bus drivers. Some prohibit driving by persons who use insulin, although those using diet or oral hypoglycemic agents are not restricted. Recently, a large city public transit system prohibited insulin-dependent diabetics from driving passenger-carrying vehicles. By a strange quirk of fate, one streetcar driver, displaced because he required insulin, was reassigned as a chauffeur, driving the automobile of the director of the transportation system. Apparently the director considered him a good risk for himself if not for the paying passengers. Many prohibitive regulations are a result of medicolegal fears.

Certain other occupations are not recommended for insulin-using diabetics. These include work on scaffolding at great heights or with high-tension wires. An insulin reaction may be hazardous to the employee and to others. Piloting jet airplanes is also forbidden to persons who require insulin or oral agents. This ruling, while discouraging to some diabetics, is understandable.

On the positive side, the young diabetic should be encouraged by the expansion in the "intelligent" job market, which has eliminated some of the disadvantages once suffered. Electronics, computer programming, data processing and many other fields are now open. The United States Civil Service Commission is an example of an enlightened attitude toward diabetics. With a very few exceptions, most Civil Service jobs are open to diabetics. The new regulations state that "All diabetics who have achieved reasonable control of the condition are eligible for Federal employment with proper placement to be based on the severity of the diabetes and the medication required for control." Further information can be obtained by writing to the Medical Director of the United States Civil Service Commission, United States Civil Service Commission, Washington, D.C. 20415. Legislation, often initiated by diabetes groups, is improving job opportunities. The job situation, while far from perfect, is improving.

Financial Aid and Tax Items. Some states offer special assistance for children or even older persons with diabetes. This may be important for the diabetic who needs special care and vocational counseling or training to become employable. The diabetic should keep careful records of medications and supplies purchased, since many may be tax-deductible items. As in the case of all special medical aids, regulations vary and the diabetic should check the rules in his own locality.

Insurance. Insurance, whether life or casualty, has always been an annoying problem to diabetics. The diabetic, in preparing for the uncertainties of life, was often uninsurable. Recently several insurance companies began to insure the lives of the "best" diabetics, although they were put in a substandard class requiring high premium payments. Now insurance has become available through some, if not all, insurance companies, although often at an additional premium. Among the factors considered are age at onset of diabetes, duration of diabetes, its severity as measured by treatment required and, of course, known complications. Other unfavorable factors include overweight or a history of other medical problems. The decision is made by the insurance company's medical department, which frequently depends on information from the diabetic's personal physician. One problem with obtaining insurance is that old, outdated actuarial tables are often used.

The American Diabetes Association, through its affiliates, has made available several life insurance plans for diabetics *"at standard rates and without medical examination,"* provided the applicant is a member of one of the Association's affiliates, has been diagnosed as a diabetic since 1958, is free of heart or kidney complications, and is under medical care with periodic examinations. There is also a plan that offers life insurance to diabetics at age 15 at "very favorable rates." These are important steps; since insurance companies are competitive, hopefully the trend will spread. Obtaining hospitalization insurance has been even more difficult than obtaining life insurance, but recently a supplemental hospital indemnity plan with relatively low group premiums for in-hospital benefits has been developed for diabetics. Employment by a sizable company or other organization that has group insurance is the best and easiest way for a person with diabetes to secure hospital coverage. Since these data change constantly, a person with diabetes should check with his own diabetes association or group.

identification cards and bracelets

All diabetics should understand the need for carrying identification concerning their diabetes. Some diabetics carry cards while others rightly prefer bracelets with an inscribed message. Unconsciousness may result for many reasons, and the diabetic should be instantly identified so that a low blood glucose reaction may be treated immediately. Sometimes diabetics with hypoglycemia are mistaken as being intoxicated and, despite protests, lose time being arrested instead of being given the needed carbohydrate. Identification cards may be obtained from the American Diabetes Association or your diabetes clinic (*Fig. 33*). The Medic Alert Foundation International of Turlock, California (*Fig. 34*) makes up bracelets,

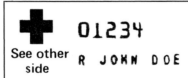
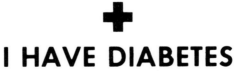

+ 01234

See other
side   R JOHN DOE

JOSLIN CLINIC IDENTIFICATION CARD

15 JOSLIN RD.   CLINIC (617) 232-8280
BOSTON, MASS. 02215   APPOINTMENTS (617) 232-4111

+

I HAVE DIABETES

If I am found unconscious, send me IMMEDIATELY to a hospital.

If I am behaving abnormally, my condition probably is the result of an overdose of INSULIN.
Give orange-juice, coca-cola, gingerale or sugar by mouth. An improvement in my behavior should result within 15 minutes.

FIG. 33. Example of an identification card for diabetics.

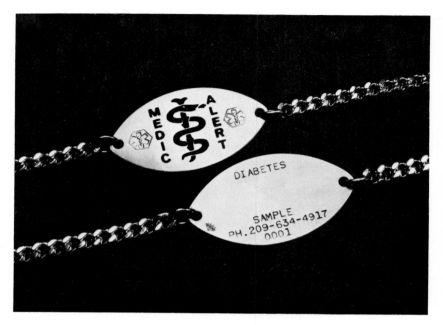

FIG. 34. A Medic Alert bracelet. For a single low fee, the Medic Alert Foundation International provides a wallet card and a bracelet or necklace engraved with the patient's medical condition(s), a membership number, and a telephone number of the Emergency Answering Service, which can provide immediate computerized medical information about the patient. Contact Medic Alert Foundation International, Turlock, California 95380.

necklaces and anklets engraved with medical information. There is no excuse for any diabetic to be without identification.

operating automobiles, boats, other vehicles

Today, driving an automobile is not a luxury, but a means of making a living. It calls for special precautions on the part of the diabetic. The same cautions apply to power boats, motorcycles or snowmobiles, among other potentially harmful vehicles. The operation of automobiles by diabetics has come increasingly under surveillance of state licensing authorities. The federal government is involved where interstate travel is concerned, as with trucks or trains. However, driving regulations vary with each state, but most require identification of the diabetic on the license application. Some states pose bizarre, poorly worded questions such as "Do you ever have fits or fainting spells?" No diabetic should ever drive without a readily available snack such as sugar or candy. Never should a diabetic skip or delay a meal while driving. An accident, even though caused by low blood glucose, is still the responsibility of the driver. Diabetics must be especially careful because, if they have poor driving records, legislatures and registries of motor vehicles may restrict their driving privileges as a group. Such regulations are becoming more commonplace with growing public concern about auto casualties. The regulations concerning boats and other powered pleasure vehicles are ill-defined as yet, but insulin reactions are no less dangerous when using these vehicles.

exercise and sports

This subject, while generally discussed earlier, is repeated to encourage diabetics who can and do participate in nearly all sports. Football players have played professionally in spite of diabetes. Bobby Clarke, one of the great hockey players, has long-term diabetes of youthful onset; he uses a sizable dose of insulin daily. Other well-known diabetic athletes include Hamilton Richardson and Bill Talbert of tennis fame; Ron Santo, the baseball player; championship skiers and indeed players in every category. The main danger is the possibility of low blood sugar reactions. Injuries pose no greater risks for diabetics than for nondiabetics, but coaches and teammates should be aware of the diabetes. Extra carbohydrate must be used as needed. After discussion with the physician, it may be possible to lower the insulin dosage on days of games or heavy exercise.

the drinking diabetic

In a physiologic sense, no physician can ever say that significant drinking is beneficial for anyone, diabetic or nondiabetic. The problem is that drinking has become a common social and business custom nearly worldwide. The late Dr. Elliott P. Joslin was adamant against the use of alcohol in any form although, with his wry sense of mischief, he confessed to sometimes allowing "patients over the age of 90" to indulge themselves just a bit. In a previous edition of this Manual he stated, "I think it far easier for a diabetic to exercise self-restraint without the use of alcohol than with it. It is certainly not needed in the diabetic dietary."

In spite of these admonitions, alcohol drinking by diabetics to one degree or another has become a fact of life. Gin is no longer necessarily equated with sin and all who drink are not inebriated. Many diabetics, attempting to live what they consider a "normal" life, will occasionally drink regardless of advice to the contrary. In any event they must understand the use and abuse of drinking.

Effects of Alcohol on the Body. Among its actions, alcohol injures the body by acting like an astringent on the cells. On the surface, alcohol cools the skin by evaporation, but in the body, it irritates mucous membranes and the stomach lining. Gastritis often occurs in the stomachs of constant drinkers. After drinking, alcohol is absorbed rapidly directly into the bloodstream from the stomach. The rest goes to the small intestine, where it is rapidly absorbed. The longer it is delayed in leaving the stomach, the slower it will be absorbed, which is why drinking with food is less intoxicating than drinking on an empty stomach.

More than 90% of the alcohol that enters the body is completely metabolized, mostly in the liver. Since the liver is the chief detoxifying organ of the body, alcohol takes some of its toll there. Apparently alcohol causes some damage to liver cells, but since the liver usually can regenerate new cells to replace the damaged cells fairly rapidly, hopefully the outcome is at least a tie score! The healthy adult metabolizes alcohol at the rate of 10 cc per hour. It takes about six hours to completely metabolize the alcohol in three ordinary drinks of whiskey (about $4\frac{1}{2}$ ounces). Eventually, of course, alcoholics may develop cirrhosis of the liver. One cannot be completely protected from the effects of alcohol by eating, and liver damage depends on the total amount of alcohol consumed as well as the speed of consumption.

Alcohol is generally classified as a depressant to the central nervous system rather than as a stimulant, despite its legendary reputation to the contrary. Alcohol has an anesthetic effect on the brain. The continued ingestion of alcohol involves more of the brain's organizing ability until thinking is affected and eventually the over-alcoholized person falls asleep.

In the past, physicians sometimes prescribed whiskey because they thought it might protect cardiac patients by relieving tension and help angina by dilating small blood vessels, but recent research shows that alcohol decreases cardiac output. Alcohol also increases the pulse rate and after heavy drinking, irregular heart rhythms may result.

One danger for diabetics who use alcohol is that posed by low blood glucose reactions. When a diabetic drinks, the liver's ability to create new glucose (gluconeogenesis) can be almost completely blocked. In the presence of alcohol, competition for the liver enzymes stops this process. Since sugar is not freely available when needed, the hypoglycemia that follows can be quite profound and prolonged, and the effects of insulin or other blood glucose lowering measures can be intensified. Also, drinking can mask the usual signals of low blood sugar. There are also more practical considerations, such as the danger of insulin reactions while driving, which have been discussed previously.

Alcohol may pose a problem for diabetics being treated with sulfonylurea-type oral agents, since the combination sometimes causes an intense flushing of the face because of surface blood vessel engorgement.

Caloric Production of Alcohol. In spite of its caloric production, alcohol is not a food. It furnishes no carbohydrate, protein or fat, and it is not helpful in nutrition. Nevertheless, 1 gram of alcohol yields 7 calories, so that it is a fuel that is used readily. The amount of alcohol in a drink is determined by the "proof." One-half of the proof represents the percentage of alcohol in a drink. For example, 80-proof whiskey contains 40% alcohol. One ounce of straight whiskey contains about 85 calories. A person who drinks alcohol adds a significant number of calories to his diet. Adding sweetened liquids, such as ginger ale or cocktail mixes, and the usual hors d'oeuvres add still more calories.

The alcohol content of beer averages about 4% in the

United States and as high as 12% in other parts of the world. Beer also contains a little more than 4% sugar and 0.6% protein. Overall, beer provides about 14 calories per ounce or about 150 calories per 12-ounce can or bottle! Some noncarbohydrate beers are sold as "dietetic" beers; they have only half as many calories but often contain more alcohol.

Wines vary greatly from high-caloric fortified wines to dry table wines, which are lower both in sugar and alcoholic content. Since wine is often consumed with meals, the probability of lowered blood glucose levels is less. "Dry" wines, such as sauternes, are probably safest for diabetics. Sherry, although "dry," still provides about 30 calories an ounce. Burgandies are difficult to judge because the manufacturers sometimes add a sugar solution to help the fermentation process. Some sparkling wines may have a lower sugar content.

Liqueurs have high carbohydrate values and should be avoided by diabetics. A list of calories contained in alcoholic beverages *without the addition of any mixers* is given in *Table 21.*

In summary, alcohol in every form, even without mixers, yields an abundance of calories with little nutritional value, if any. The harder spirits such as whiskeys have a high alcohol content and provide more calories than, for example, unsweetened wines. Alcohol is prohibited in most weight-reduction diets because, in a 1200-calorie daily diet, one drink may contain 10% of the daily intake. Since alcohol is very easily burned as fuel but has no lasting food value, the drinker is caught on the horns of a dilemma. If he does not eat while drinking, the alcohol is absorbed at a faster rate and, if he does not become intoxicated, he might still have a low blood glucose reaction. On the other hand, if a person drinks and eats considerably, the caloric intake is great and the food is more likely to be stored for the future in unflattering places such as the classic "beer belly."

Obviously, it is best for the diabetic not to drink, but if he does drink, it should be done sparingly and intelligently. A drink with an ounce-and-a-half of whiskey should preferably be consumed with water, soda or "on the rocks" as a before-dinner drink when at home or at a social function with friends. Although there is no carbohydrate in such drinks, they are generally considered as a "carbohydrate exchange," because this is the simplest way of measuring the calories. In

TABLE 21. Amounts of Carbohydrate, Alcohol, and Calories
            in Alcoholic Drinks

Alcoholic Drinks	Household Measure	Total Grams	Grams of Carbo-hydrate*	Grams of Alcohol†	Calories (Approx.)
Whiskey: bourbon, Irish, rye, and Scotch	1 brandy glass (1 oz.)	30	none	10½–12	75–85
Brandy, gin and rum	1 brandy glass (1 oz.)	30	none	10½–13	17–90
Liqueurs and cordials	1 cordial glass (⅔ oz.)	20	4–10	4–7	50–80
Malt liquors: ale, beer, porter, and stout	1 glass (8 oz.)	240	7–14	7–14	80–150
Wines:					
Sweet, domestic	1 wine glass (3½ oz.)	100	8–14	13–15	140–165
Sweet, imported	1 wine glass (3½ oz.)	100	3–20	10½–18	110–175
Dry, domestic	1 wine glass (3½ oz.)	100	½–4	10–11	75–90
Dry, imported	1 wine glass (3½ oz.)	100	½–3	8–14	60–110
Cider:					
Sweet	1 glass (8 oz.)	240	25	trace	100
Hard (fermented)	1 wine glass (3½ oz.)	100	1	5	40

*Every gram of carbohydrate supplies four calories.
†Every gram of alcohol supplies seven calories.
Use of alcoholic beverages should be discussed with your physician.

theory, especially if a diabetic has a weight problem, the
equivalent amount of carbohydrate should be deducted from
the meal. The physician is not nearly as concerned about the
patient who drinks rarely or occasionally or may have a glass
of champagne at his daughter's wedding as he is concerned
about the person who habitually drinks "socially." In the
United States, this can be a significant amount. Drinking

234 LIVING WITH DIABETES

should be discussed with your own physician. Obviously, Dr. Elliott Joslin's admonition "DON'T!" is the best advice for anyone, especially the person with diabetes. On the other hand, astute diabetics who drink intelligently may do so with a minimum of difficulty or risk to themselves.

smoking

Physicians may differ in their advice about drinking for diabetics, but they are almost unanimously opposed to smoking for everyone, especially diabetics. While some physicians find it difficult to be as forceful as they might on the subject, recently a health authority said, "We must appreciate the obvious fact that the time and effort spent by physicians in convincing their patients not to smoke cigarettes will produce more meaningful and useful years of life than all the cardiac transplants have produced." The increased risks of cancer and emphysema for the smoker in the general population are well known. For diabetics, the fact that their risk of cardiovascular complications is greater should be an added deterrent to smoking. Tobacco smoking is thought to increase constriction of the smaller blood vessels, further impeding circulation. Older persons as well as long-duration diabetics often have decreased circulation in their extremities, so for them, smoking may add insult to injury. Since smoking is a most difficult habit to break, people best avoid this struggle by not starting. As to the number of cigarettes required to cause damage, it is impossible to say that six cigarettes daily won't and 20 will. There is no way to determine the precise danger point. Especially for diabetics, the number of daily cigarettes permitted should be *none.*

the drug culture

The use of "hard" drugs (cocaine, heroin and morphine) is definitely prohibited. In addition to being illegal, the use of all of these drugs is harmful and indeed potentially lethal—they are mentioned here only for emphasis. The drugs commonly used have a physical as well as mental addictive power that cannot be underestimated. They are dangerous; their effects are not predictable from person to person. While the relationships of these drugs to crime, mental deterioration and physical illness may seem to be contradicted in news reports occasionally, such a relationship should be more believed than disbelieved. One problem is that, while nearly everyone condemns the so-called hard drugs, they tend to take a softer line about amphetamines (speed) and marijuana (pot). Fortunately, LSD has fallen from grace because of incontrovertible evidence of its harm.

It is difficult to understand the apparently benign condemnation or even toleration of both amphetamines and marijuana in the permissive cultural atmosphere of today by others than the law enforcement agencies. Both of these drugs have the potential for harm, and vary from the "hard" drugs in degree and speed of attainment of harm. Because of prescribing restrictions, amphetamine is becoming difficult to obtain for even those few medical situations where it might be useful. Marijuana, on the other hand, is still generally unlawful, although laws against possession of small amounts are being amended. Amphetamine is ineffective as an appetite suppressor for any length of time. It does speed up reaction time and gives a feeling of great ability, but intolerance to it develops and more is needed to achieve the same effect. Research shows that amphetamines can increase the breakdown of glycogen from the liver; the net result is the need for increased insulin requirement in many patients. Personality changes and depression are only a few of the long-term problems that can follow the use of amphetamines.

It is more difficult to be dogmatic about the marijuana question, especially since legislatures are "decriminalizing" the possession of small amounts of "pot" for personal use. Some studies have given marijuana a relatively clean bill of health. It is a stimulant and a mild hallucinogen made from the flower tops or leaves of the female hemp plant (*Cannabis sativa*). The chief active ingredient is tetrahydrocannabinol. It is usually smoked but may be sniffed or swallowed. Initial effects are usually euphoria, mood swings, loss of inhibitions and changes in time and space relationships lasting from two to four hours. Long-term use may result in an apathy and lack of interest that has been called a "drop-out syndrome." This is seen frequently in the Middle East where usage is common. Other adverse effects can be panic or psychotic reactions and psychologic dependence. A true "high" interferes with the performance of many complex skills. Some researchers report electrocardiographic changes and lowered testosterone levels. Marijuana is thought to weaken the body's immune system. This list of harmful effects seems endless, but is not without its challengers, since many of the studies supporting such claims were poorly designed. The arguments about the use of pot leading to harder drugs are not substantiated. However, the possession of significant amounts and use are still illegal in varying degrees.

For the diabetic, additional problems arise with the use of marijuana. For one thing, marijuana may mask hypoglycemic reactions. It also is reported to have caused increased breakdown in glycogen with increased insulin requirements. A bad characteristic is the reported craving for sweets or other foods among pot users. This craving has been given many names, including the "hungries" or the "munchies." Perhaps the most damaging indictment against the use of marijuana is the fact that users of marijuana are usually seeking escape into unreality. The diabetic already has a handicap: he must compete in an increasingly difficult and competitive world. No one says, "since you are diabetic, we will make it easier for you." Anything the diabetic does to foster a sense of unreality, to limit the ability to focus his thoughts or to increase the tendency to "cop out," adds to his problems. It is like tying weights around one's legs in a foot race. The argument that harm from the use of marijuana has not been completely proven is not a plausible defense for its use. Tobacco was considered to be a safe and pleasant diversion for some 300 years before its hazards became known. Can anyone guarantee that marijuana will have a completely clean bill of health in the near future or even 100 years from now?

Many legitimate drugs can be badly used. For example, drugs in the "sleeping pill" and tranquilizer categories can lead to dependence and the need for stronger medications with occasional tragic results. Their use in combination with alcohol is especially dangerous.

medications the diabetic may use

The diabetic can use almost any medication that nondiabetics use. Exceptions would be medications that use highly sweetened or concentrated syrups for a base. Cortisone raises blood glucose levels and is used only by direction of the physician; when required for illness, cortisone can be used with proper adjustment of insulin dosage as needed.

Patients sometimes are concerned about medicines such as those used for symptomatic relief of colds. These may have labels that state, "Not to be used in case of hypertension, diabetes . . . ." These medicines often contain minute amounts of drugs that have an adrenalin-like action; they tend to raise blood sugar levels, although usually very slightly, if at all. The warning is a simple legal one, much like a sign reading "Road officially closed." Yet, with care, the road can often be safely traveled. The purpose is to protect the highway authorities from real or imagined responsibility. Similarly, the drug warning may be overlooked if the patient's physician indicates that the medication is safe when judiciously used. Most medications that may cause difficulties are obtained by physician's prescription only. Of course, there may be specific drug warnings from time to time, such as the alleged relationship between *the use of tranquilizers and possible birth defects* if used during the first three months of pregnancy. However, these warnings apply to diabetics and nondiabetics alike.

Other Problem Medications.   Birth control pills may slightly elevate blood glucose levels, but this would be a concern only for the borderline diabetic. The question of possible detrimental long-term effects from the use of birth control pills is still being debated. These dangers, however, are the same for diabetics and nondiabetics. Cortisone and cortisone-like drugs, as noted, may antagonize the effect of insulin. Epinephrine (Adrenalin) raises the blood glucose level. Diuretics (used to remove excess fluid from the body) impair glucose tolerance in many diabetics. Other problems may arise from medications that tend to decrease blood sugar levels either by their own action or by potentiating medications used for this purpose. The effects of alcohol, aspirin and anticoagulants (such as Coumadin) in this regard have been discussed earlier.

In conclusion, since one medication may interfere with or increase the action of another, it is important to consult your physician when taking several medications.

surgery and diabetes

Today, with proper preparation and care of diabetes, any necessary surgical operations can be performed on the diabetic. If the diabetes has been neglected, it may be necessary to postpone the surgical procedure long enough to bring the diabetes under better regulation in order to ensure the best results. However, with preparation and monitoring, even the most complex procedures are now done in those with diabetes.

dental problems

The dental complications of diabetes, while often not specific, are such that dentists sometimes suspect diabetes because of the poor condition of the teeth and gums. More particularly, uncontrolled diabetes seems to accentuate disease of the gums (periodontal disease), which is the second most common cause for the loss of teeth. Certainly conditions like hereditary changes and poor general mouth care may precede the diabetes and influence some of the problems. However, when diabetes is grossly uncontrolled, it appears that patients lose their teeth at a faster rate (perhaps even a decade earlier) than they should. Additional problems in the mouth that may accompany an uncontrolled diabetic state are increased incidence of fungus infection and possibly poor healing.

acupuncture

With renewed interest in the People's Republic of China, there has been widespread interest in acupuncture, and many diabetics have hoped that this technique might solve some of their problems. Unfortunately, there are few well-researched studies on the subject; it is not well-documented, even in China. Acupuncture is based on a theory of flowing nerve energy and the release of nerve impulses. It has been used mostly for the treatment of pain or as an anesthetic. There is no evidence that acupuncture is useful in the treatment of diabetes, and if it causes the diabetic to neglect accepted treatment, it could indeed be harmful and should be avoided.

contact lenses

Diabetics are beset by many problems that may be considered minor to everyone else but major to them. Many are concerned about the use of contact lenses. In general, if the outside of the eye is healthy and if the lenses are well-fitted by an expert, they can be used by diabetics. Hard corneal lenses, soft corneal lenses and scleral lenses are available. Patients who may be subject to unconsciousness may be good candidates for soft lenses, but anyone who may be subject to periods of difficult diabetes regulation, such as pregnant women in the early stages of pregnancy, should wait until their diabetes has stabilized after the period before being fitted for contact lenses. Diabetics with healthy eyes probably can use contact lenses, if expertly fitted; because of the diabetic's increased susceptibility to infection, lenses should be rechecked at intervals.

ear piercing

Another common question concerns the diabetic's wish to have her ears pierced. Usually, a small hole is punched through the ear lobe and wires or studs are inserted immediately. Upon healing, a permanent canal exists for use with better grades of earrings. If the procedure is skillfully done with proper precaution against infection, the diabetic should be able to enjoy the popular pierced earrings even as do her nondiabetic sisters.

camps for diabetics

Special camps for youngsters with diabetes are now widely available. Certainly the young diabetic has unique problems, both physiologic and especially psychologic. Young diabetics from the ages of 8 to 16 (the most popular years for camping) have unique problems that can be greatly helped with a camping situation (see page 210).

marriage and childbearing

Dr. Joslin once wrote, "It is a great advantage for a diabetic to be married because of the intimate protection and care thereby obtained." However, as he also pointed out, certain matters must be faced by the diabetic and the nondiabetic partner. Sometimes medical information is sought from the physician by a young diabetic contemplating marriage. Generally, such discussions should be conducted with both partners present.

Marriage Counselling. Marriage counselling, in general, is widely sought and frequently ignored. The desire to marry and have children is natural and universal. One of the more urgent questions asked by the future diabetic parent is, "Will my children have diabetes?" The hereditary aspects of diabetes have been discussed earlier. There are other important considerations in marriage.

Marriage to a person with any chronic condition poses problems that require patience and understanding. What may be an intolerable burden to some marriage partners may be no problem to others. Although facts and data usually do little to change minds where human emotions are involved, the person contemplating marriage to a diabetic should consider the following factors. (1) The possibility of complications that may occur after a period of years must be considered. Disability or premature death may occur—not necessarily, but possibly. (2) The chances of a female diabetic having a stillborn baby are greater than those of nondiabetic women, even though this risk has been appreciably lessened. Also, even though the number may be small, congenital defects are more frequent in children born to diabetic mothers. (3) The nondiabetic partner must realize that the nature of diabetes requires medical supervision throughout life and that there is at present no "cure." (4) Special problems with employment and insurance may arise.

It would seem that the negative aspects of marriage have been stressed unnecessarily. There are many favorable features as well and, if all the facts are known, the partners may establish a background for a stable and happy marriage. The facts, however, must be faced squarely by both partners.

Some Practical Aspects of Married Life. One aspect of marriage that is not discussed often enough with diabetic patients is sex. People often seek advice from those who know even less than they. Diabetics have the same sex characteristics and desires as others. When able to perform sexual pursuits normally, diabetics usually have no problems with fertility. The difficulties, if any, concern the eventual inability of the diabetic male to have a "normal" sex life. "Normal" is a very difficult term to define. Even nondiabetics vary tremendously in sex drive and ability. Some males begin to taper off after age 40 while others may perform acceptably after age 70.

In general, the situation may be summarized as follows. The sexual drive and performance of the diabetic woman seem unimpaired. The possible problems of the diabetic man have been looked at in the past decade or so and the following facts seem evident. While diabetic men are subject to the same tensions and resultant lack of performance as nondiabetic men, an additional problem seems to occur in about a quarter of middle-aged diabetic men. These men seem to lack sexual potency unrelated to degree of diabetic control or duration of diabetes. The decline in function is steady and appears unrelated to sexual interest or libido. Certainly, psychologic problems of any type, including sexual concern and the use of alcohol and even other medications can compound the situation. A search for these factors and the avoidance of useless as well as expensive medications is important to men with this problem. Furthermore, counselling both husband and wife about their expectations and ways of expressing intimate feelings is another avenue of help for these couples. Recently various appliances and surgical penile inserts have been devised and have improved the outlook for some patients.

According to present data, the impotence related to diabetes is not a hormonal lack, but mostly due to neuropathy, which may well be related to duration of diabetes and probably the degree of diabetes control. However, this is one area about which positive statements are difficult to make. It is difficult to evaluate specific treatment, since some patients respond to different types of treatment while others do not respond at all.

Pregnancy and Childbearing. The nondiabetic wives of men with diabetes have no added barrier to successful pregnancy because of the husband's condition. However, statistically, young women with diabetes do not fare quite as well or have as successful an outcome as nondiabetic women. With expert management during pregnancy, the difficulties are significantly decreased. Six per cent of all individuals with diabetes are women between the ages of 15 and 40. One per cent of all pregnant women tested for diabetes have elevated levels of blood glucose. With pregnancy, there sometimes occurs a special type of diabetes known as "gestational diabetes," in which elevated blood glucose levels may appear only during pregnancy. In half of these women, overt diabetes can be diagnosed within 15 years of their pregnancy. Pregnancy sometimes intensifies a very mild diabetes, making it more obvious. This occurs because some of the placental hormones make insulin less effective. The most important of these is a hormone, made in the placenta, which makes fat, protein and carbohydrate available to the embryo. The placenta is also believed to be capable of destroying insulin.

Diabetes changes during each three months (or trimester) of pregnancy and immediately after delivery. The diagnostic levels for blood glucose are usually higher during pregnancy than in the nonpregnant state. During the first trimester, diabetes sometimes improves and insulin requirements may decrease slightly. Insulin reactions often occur without warning, but these do not injure the fetus. Diabetes is more severe in the second trimester. Insulin requirements increase and ketoacidosis and coma can occur rather easily, endangering the life of the future baby. During the third trimester, diabetes again is severe and treatment is complicated because the kidney threshold for sugar is lower and the amount of sugar lost in the urine does not coincide with the amount of sugar in the blood. Labor is a form of exercise and reduces the insulin requirement. The insulin need drops dramatically in the first several days after delivery. The diabetes improves so much that there is almost a remission, but about five days after delivery, the same amount of insulin used before pregnancy is necessary.

Before the discovery of insulin, few women with diabetes were able to become pregnant. Some of those who did died undelivered. Today, very few diabetic women require special studies or treatment for sterility. Spontaneous abortion occurs in about 10 to 20% of all pregnancies, and this is the same as occurs in diabetes unless very many years of diabetes have gone by or complications have taken place. With modern care, most diabetic women are able to go through pregnancy, some with some difficulty. Most are successful provided that the time of delivery is selected with care on the basis of clinical judgement and the results of tests now available. On the average, the diabetic woman is delivered in the 37th or 38th week, rather than the usual 40th week of pregnancy. Obviously, superb care of the diabetes is vital.

Babies of Diabetics. Babies of diabetic mothers show some differences from babies of nondiabetic mothers. One of the commonest is a very low blood glucose level, measuring below 40 mg. per cent, often due to the increase in the baby's insulin level. Often, other chemical changes occur that are not too serious and can be managed by the physician. The well-known heavy weight of babies of diabetic mothers is due to early and excessive fat deposition. The pancreas actually shows larger islets of Langerhans with more insulin-producing cells and very few cells that produce glucagon. While sometimes congenital anomalies may occur, most are minor and others are correctable with modern-day care, and the babies grow and develop quite normally. Exceptional or unusual tests for diabetes in children of diabetic mothers are unnecessary; only an awareness of the possibilities and observation are required. Such children carry a genetic potential for diabetes, but if they ever develop diabetes, it may be years later.

Can Diabetes be Controlled During Pregnancy? The blood glucose can be kept at normal levels before meals. Urine sugar spilled in 24 hours can be kept at or below 10% of the total sugar and starch intake for the day. Small amounts of acetone without elevated urine sugar may occur after fasting during sleep. This is usually corrected with a larger bedtime snack. However, acetone with elevated urine sugar levels indicates a need for larger amounts of insulin.

Young women with diabetes must take the very best care of the condition at all times, but particularly during pregnancy. Excellent care in the years before marriage and childbearing increases the chances that living, healthy offspring will be born. Studies of children of diabetic mothers are important.

The chance of developing frank diabetes under age 20 in these children is under 10%, although some will show an increased glucose tolerance test. This is also true if the father has diabetes.

Present results of pregnancy in diabetics show that, with good care, the unwanted excessive fluid can be decreased and premature deliveries are less frequent. When fetuses are alive at "viability" (the 28th week), 90% can be delivered successfully and survive in a healthy state, as compared to 97% in the general population.

Birth Control. In general, women with diabetes may use the same birth control measures as those without diabetes. The oral contraceptive medications have the same contraindications (circumstances in which their use is not advised) for both groups of women and this should be discussed with one's gynecologist or general practitioner. Besides the general problems of risk versus possible gain with the oral contraceptive pills, there are additional considerations for diabetic women. First, diabetic control can be worsened in patients who do not have obvious insulin-dependent diabetes at the time when they begin to take the pills. For example, a woman whose diabetes is controlled by the use of oral hypoglycemic agents or diet alone may find that her diabetes can be accentuated with the prolonged use of pregnancy-simulating hormones. This should be a consideration in prescribing the "pill" for many adult-onset diabetic patients. Secondly, the incidence of uterine cancer in women in the 50- to 60-year age group appears to be higher in diabetic and hypertensive women. Therefore, the use of hormones for whatever reason should be kept to a minimum during these years. In general, most physicians do not prescribe the oral contraceptive pills for longer than five years totally in any particular woman's life span. This should also be a good rule for diabetic women. Recent research has centered around the development of long-duration injectable agents to prevent pregnancy.

Intrauterine devices have gained in popularity, although there is some question about their possible relationship to infection or cancer at the site of insertion. Clearly, the use of these devices requires close observation by a physician. Newer types of contraceptive agents are also under investigation. Meanwhile, long-used forms of birth control, such as condoms, diaphragms, spermicidal jelly and fertility rhythm methods, are still used widely. Clearly, there is no one perfect form of contraception. Physician and patient should consider whether a particular contraceptive method or pregnancy itself represents the greater risk. Increasingly, birth control is being achieved by vasectomy in the male. In this simple, safe procedure, part of the ducts that conduct sperm is excised. In the female, the ligation (tying off) of the Fallopian tubes has enjoyed increasing popularity. These surgical procedures do not impair sexual function. In fact, freedom of the fear of pregnancy sometimes improves sexual performance.

the older diabetic

There is a tendency to believe that the diabetes of the older person is free of difficulties. This is not necessarily true. Although their diabetes is often not as unstable as that of juveniles, these patients may suffer the same acute complications of diabetes that befall others. A problem may arise from the fact that, in the older person, the threshold at which sugar appears in the urine may be much higher than normal, so that the blood sugar level may be 250 or 300 mg. per cent with little or no urine sugar. This is deceptive, and during infections the blood sugar may rise still higher to levels of impending acidosis without the patient's awareness. Many older diabetics are chronically undertreated and have consistently elevated blood sugar levels. This may be accompanied by dehydration, with the possible development of hyperosmolar acidosis, a dangerous condition related to dehydration.

The older patient is a potential candidate for foot problems caused by diminished circulation. Kidney function is not as effective and ingested medications tend to remain in the body longer than expected. Because of this, the longer-acting oral hypoglycemic agents may cause very low blood sugar levels. Severe insulin reactions are also likely to be more serious in older persons, and it may be wiser to permit a modest elevation of blood glucose levels in order to avoid such episodes in patients whose cerebral circulation is often decreased.

Diet can be another problem. With limited social lives and friendships, some older persons have poor nutrition. Too often the woman who has cooked for a whole family for most of her life fails to prepare adequate meals for herself when she is alone. Many such people live on toast, soups, tea or foods that require a minimum of preparation. The craving for sweets often increases. Poor dentures may add to the dietary inadequacies. Projects such as Meals-on-Wheels may help to ensure good nutrition for the older patient.

traveling with diabetes

Each year the world becomes smaller and thousands of people who never traveled before go to faraway places. There is no reason why those with diabetes should not be among them. Most of the comforts and conveniences of home can now be found even in remote places, and the jet age has permitted our prejudices to travel with us. An Oriental adage states that the best of all worlds consists of "a Chinese cook, a Japanese wife and American plumbing!" If diabetes is well-controlled at home, travel should not be burdensome. However, if the diabetic has difficulty controlling his condition under ideal home circumstances, the uncertainties of travel can cause further difficulties. Very unstable diabetics who have insulin reactions without warning should endeavor to get their condition as stable as possible before leaving. It may be best to travel with a knowledgeable companion.

Before Leaving. It is almost impossible to begin preparing too early for a trip. After the itinerary has been chosen and passports, visas and tickets obtained, the detailed planning starts. It is important to make certain that the health insurance policy applies to the areas that will be visited. Inoculations should be brought up to date as needed. The regulations concerning smallpox vaccinations have changed recently, so they are no longer required. The tourist returning to the United States no longer has to show his yellow vaccination card unless he has been in an area where yellow fever has been reported in the last six days, or smallpox in the last 14 days. However, smallpox has not been reported in this country in the last 20 years and is no longer a worldwide threat. In fact, the World Health Organization has announced that, for all practical purposes, smallpox has been eradicated, although some countries still demand evidence of vaccination. Vaccinations last for three years, and revaccination does not carry even the very low risk for complications that occurs with the initial vaccination. Yellow fever, poliomyelitis and typhoid are endemic in some parts of the world, as are infectious hepatitis, tetanus and cholera. Information concerning these diseases can be obtained from the local health department, the U.S. Public Health Service or the Communicable Disease Center in Atlanta, Georgia. The pamphlet, "Immunization Information for International Travel," can be obtained from the Superintendent of Documents, U.S. Government Printing Office, Washington, D.C. 20402.

A stay in commonly visited centers in Europe poses no problem. When planning travel in Asia, Africa, Central or South America, it is wise to consult your physician about other inoculations. Protection against cholera and infectious hepatitis is short in duration, but protection against the other diseases lasts for reasonably long periods. In many parts of the world, malaria also is a continuous problem. It is now possible to take a preventive medication at weekly intervals for several weeks before and after the trip, which reduces the chances of acquiring malaria.

Choosing Clothes.   Like everyone else, diabetics often take too many clothes when traveling. However, because they must watch their feet scrupulously, they should tuck in an extra pair of walking shoes. Most foreigners walk more than we do—and walking is always in style. *Simple baggage tip:* put a large initial with adhesive tape on the side of each piece of baggage. When the modern jumbo jet with 300 passengers unloads with 900 pieces of brown, blue or gray baggage, they all look alike. This simple tip may help you to spot yours more quickly.

Health Record and Identification.   It is useful to carry a note from your physician stating your current medical condition and listing medications by their *generic* rather than trade names (which vary all over the world). For example, list tolbutamide instead of Orinase (also known as Artosin, Rastinon and other names—see Appendix 9). The generic name is understood nearly everywhere.

Diabetes identification is important at home and even more vital while traveling abroad. Although diabetics generally have no particular problems at customs, an identification card or bracelet may also be useful in placating a dubious official who may cast a baleful eye on the supply of syringes and needles! If you take insulin, the physician's certificate should also include a statement regarding the need for syringes and needles.

Personal Medication.   For most trips, it is best to bring necessary medicines with you. An extra syringe and needle can be carried in alcohol in a rubber-capped container, although most diabetics who travel now use disposable syringe and needle combinations. Travel packs of alcohol swabs are available. Any prescribed medicines should be brought along with some aspirin and foot powder to complete the package. Make certain that you have a few days' supply of needed medicines and insulin with you in your hand or flight bag. There is always the possibility that checked-through baggage may inadvertently go to a destination other than yours. Although insulin is obtainable nearly all over the world, foreign labels may be confusing. The brands most readily available are shown in Appendix 6. Do not worry about refrigeration for insulin. It can tolerate the same temperatures as you for several weeks or months. Take enough insulin with you to last for most trips.

Urine Testing While Traveling.   Most travelers prefer strip tests, such as Diastix, Clinistix or Tes-Tape, or Clinitest tablets. Foil-wrapped Clinitest tablets are slightly more expensive than those sold in bulk form, but are worth the difference in cost because they travel better. As at home, urine tests that continuously read $3+$ and $4+$ should lead to testing for acetone. Except in emergencies, urine testing should be sufficient for most trips.

Up, Up, Away!   Most international travel now is done by jet airplane. This is the fastest and the best way for diabetics to travel because it is less disrupting to the schedule. Fly during daylight hours when possible. When arriving in the late afternoon or evening, it is easier to maintain the usual diabetes schedule as well as getting a good night's rest. Changes in time can upset the internal clock that governs eating and sleeping and keeps other body functions running smoothly. Most people need a day after a major jet trip to get back into a normal rhythm. If possible, nothing important should be scheduled on the day after arrival. Most well-versed diabetics have no trouble in choosing a satisfactory meal from airline foods. Many airlines provide special diets if these are requested in advance when the reservations are made. A few airlines will honor a written menu recommended by your physician. If the diabetes is very unstable, the stewardess should be reminded of your condition so that if you require something sweet in a hurry or if there is a delay in serving, you can have some priority. The chances are great that things will go well.

Time Zones. While the speed of a jet shortens trips, it also shortens the day going east or lengthens the day going west (*Fig. 35*). For example, flying east from New York to Paris shortens the day by six hours. Going west from New York to Hawaii, the day is very much longer. When returning to the United States from Europe, it is possible to get daytime flights, but flying to Europe from the East Coast almost surely involves a night flight. Diabetics worry about insulin adjustments. Most often the west-east flight disturbs them. Most flights to Europe start at an hour of the night when the diabetic has already had his evening meal. About an hour after takeoff, a meal is usually served. After a short sleep, the traveler is landing in Europe at perhaps 10 a.m. when it would be 4 a.m. at home. The person who takes less than 20 units of insulin daily will probably have no problems, but larger insulin doses tend to overlap. This may be avoided by lowering the insulin dose on the day of arrival by the portion of the day lost. For example, since you lose 25% of a day en route to London and you take 40 units of NPH, the insulin dose should be 30 units or 25% less. This applies especially to the intermediate (NPH or Lente) insulins. If you take clear insulin as well, you may be able to eliminate it the first day if the tests are negative. Persons who take blood-sugar-lowering tablets are less likely to have problems. However, if such tablets are taken twice daily and the urine tests are sugar-free, it may be possible to skip the first dose on arrival. On the long day flying west, the urine tests may show glucose and you may need an extra dose of clear insulin upon arrival. Your physician can advise you about other methods of adjusting medications. North and south travel poses no problems because few time zones are crossed.

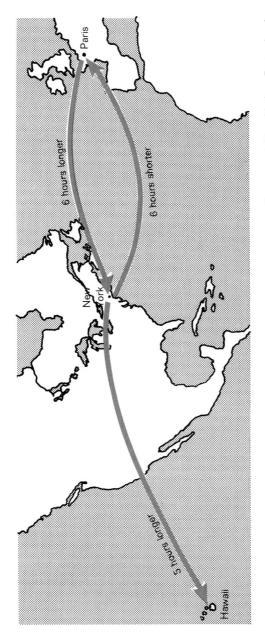

FIG. 35. When traveling, the day becomes shorter going east and longer going west. Going *east*, New York to Paris, the day is six hours shorter; Hawaii to New York, five hours shorter. Going *west*, Paris to New York, the day is six hours longer; New York to Hawaii, five hours longer. Flying north or south doesn't make much difference, because generally one crosses only one time zone.

Problems en Route. The chances of low blood sugar reactions occurring while flying are minimal because there is little activity and large amounts of food are served. Airsickness is rare but medication, if needed, will be useful only if taken *before* it is needed. If susceptible, have your physician prescribe meclizine (Bonine), dimenhydrinate (Dramamine) or cyclizine (Marezine). Passengers should occasionally walk up and down the aisle to avoid possible blood clotting in the legs caused by inflammation of the veins; this is called "passenger phlebitis." This may result from continuously sitting with the seat pressing on the backs of the knees. Most jet planes are now pressurized to 5,000 or 6,000 feet or lower no matter how high they fly. While it is possible to pressurize planes to sea level, it would be impractical because of the extensive equipment and thickening of the airplane shell that would be necessary. A person aboard the plane should be able to breathe as well as he does on land. Passengers should drink water or other liquids frequently to offset the dehydrating effects of air conditioning aboard airplanes.

Travel by Ship. While the number of transoceanic crossings by ship is decreasing, the relaxed life of a cruise may tempt the diabetic. Most large cruise ships have competent medical staffs and some have hospitals. Although there are no problems with time zones, never was a ship built that didn't pitch and roll during stormy weather, especially on the North Atlantic. Seasickness, for the nondiabetic, means a temporary inconvenience and a few missed meals, but for the diabetic, an extended gastrointestinal upset can be a real problem. The remedies previously mentioned to prevent motion sickness can help, but they are not foolproof. Unless you are sure of smooth, sheltered sailing or know yourself to be a good sailor no matter what the seas, jet plane travel is the least disrupting means of travel.

On Arriving. Avoid overeating, overdrinking and overexerting, especially on the first day. Your "travel cycle" may not have caught up with you. The food and drinking water are usually quite safe in the major hotels in the developed countries. However, while the water may not contain dangerous organisms, it may differ from the water to which you are accustomed. Generally, in most hotels and certainly away, it is safest to use bottled water. Cooked foods are usually safe in accepted hotels and restaurants. Be cautious with foods away from ordinary tourist centers and avoid raw food unless you have peeled it yourself. Generally, the hotel that caters to foreign visitors is the safest place to eat.

"Tourista"—the Curse of the Traveler. Not much is known about the very annoying condition known as "tourista," "Montezuma's revenge" and other exotic names. This illness, usually not serious, is characterized by abdominal cramping, diarrhea, nausea, and at times, chills and low-grade fever, usually lasting only one to a few days. In only a few cases is a definite bacterial organism found. For United States visitors, it most commonly occurs in the Mediterranean areas, Asia and some parts of Central and South America. The cause is not always known, although recent studies suggest that bacteria may be responsible. There are no satisfactory preventive measures except good sense and caution. After diarrhea develops, a bland diet consisting of tea, rice and clear soup is usually adequate although the diabetic must remember to use sweetened food or liquids to make certain that the carbohydrate intake is adequate. Any number of medications, such as Kaopectate or Lomotil, can be prescribed in advance by your physician and taken along for use in case of need. Antibiotics are rarely needed unless the condition persists more than a couple of days, in which case it is best to see a physician.

How to Find a Physician. First of all, your own doctor may know of physicians abroad. In addition, many countries have diabetes associations affiliated with the International Diabetes Federation (10, Queen Anne Street, London W1 M 0BD). They or the American Diabetes Association (600 Fifth Ave., New York, N.Y. 10020) may be contacted in advance for a list of diabetes-trained physicians in countries you will visit. Most major hotels also have access to physicians who speak English as does the United States Embassy or consulate in each country. An organization called Intermedic (777 Third Ave., New York, N.Y. 10017) lists English-speaking physicians who treat patients for a set fee. There are very few places in the world without adequate medical service, and into those very few areas only the best trained and most self-reliant diabetic should venture.

Other Hints.   As noted earlier, the insulins and other medicines most commonly used here are not only obtainable elsewhere around the world but often are made by the same companies that make them for you. If you do need to buy insulin abroad, you can show your insulin bottle to the pharmacist, who generally can find the equivalent. As noted earlier, the greatest danger to the diabetic who drives is insulin reaction. Snacks and meals *must* be taken on time or a bit sooner and something sweet should be available in the car. *Bus* or *train travel* can require advance planning because of the infrequency of the stops and the usually crowded conditions of terminals when you do stop. Carry snacks and be sure to eat when you get an opportunity. Carry insulin with you.

It is wise to carry either an extra pair of eyeglasses with you or the prescription for yours in case a pair is broken. Tourists can be very helpless if they cannot see well. If you have spare dentures, bring them. Another important thing to remember in traveling is the care of the feet—proper bathing, frequent changing of socks, treatment of athlete's foot and other minor infections. This, along with plenty of rest, can do a lot to prevent foot complications and make your trip much more enjoyable.

In summary, at home or abroad, your good diabetes training is your best friend and with that, the diabetic can happily succumb to the wanderlust that infects all of us from time to time. Have a safe and happy trip!

12

Past, Present and Future

In Charles Dickens' *A Christmas Carol,* Ebenezar Scrooge was awakened from sleep to meet the three Spirits of Christmas Past, Present, and Future. To some extent, today's diabetics are in the same situation. They have heard of the stark realities of the past. They know the present offers a tremendous improvement for them and enables them to lead useful lives. Mostly they are concerned about the future. Will things continue to improve? When will today's expanding knowledge and research efforts produce results? Will the miracles of the future arrive in time to help them?

the spirit of diabetes past

This Spirit tells a very grim story. Before the discovery of insulin, diabetics were purposely undernourished to allow them to survive. However, even then not all those with diabetes were destined for an early death. Those who had some insulin-making capabilities survived by decreasing their food intake to an absolute minimum. Stories are told about how foods were washed and rewashed to remove all vestiges of carbohydrate. Juveniles had more difficulty in surviving. Infections were a menace and those with severe infections frequently died.

Diabetic ketoacidosis and coma were the greatest hazards of all. The first volume of Dr. Elliott P. Joslin's record ledger, documenting the causes of death during the initial years of his practice in the early part of the century, was studded with the entries, "coma," "coma," "coma." Many diabetics of that day were gaunt and emaciated and had no hope for the future. Those who survived not only had good medical care by the standards of that day, but were very lucky indeed.

the spirit of diabetes present

Today the diabetic is very often a frustrated person. He understands that life is immeasurably better for diabetics than it has ever been, but he is impatient to see the new research wonders he has been promised in newspaper and magazine articles.

At present, more than 50 years after the discovery of insulin, many problems still exist. For one thing, although the injected insulins are truly miraculous, the method of delivery is still unphysiologic compared to the release of insulin by the normal pancreas. When the nondiabetic person starts to eat, substances secreted from the gastrointestinal tract alert the pancreas to start insulin secretion. As digestion continues, insulin secretion continues. The amount of insulin and the speed of release are determined by the blood glucose level and the rate of change as well as the size and composition of the meal. For this reason, the person with normal beta cells in the pancreas rarely elevates the blood glucose above 150 mg. per cent, even an hour or more after eating. The blood sugar level will remain within the normal range even after the largest of meals.

On the other hand, the diabetic using injected insulin must use the proper type and amount, taking into consideration activities planned for the next 24 hours as well as his diet. Allowances must be made for exercise, infection or stress. The diabetic and the physician must make an educated guess 24 hours or more in advance. Blood and urine sugar levels can change so rapidly that it is impossible to maintain a "normal" blood glucose at all times. Insulin as now used is far from perfect, since it is a very rare diabetic who has a normal blood glucose immediately after a meal, especially after breakfast. This is not necessarily the patient's fault. The patient very often accepts the need for intelligent meal planning. Most patients soon lose their objections to the need for daily insulin injections. What disturbs them most is the insecure feeling that they might not be getting the optimal amount of insulin when they need it. They find themselves caught between the perils of too high or too low blood glucose levels.

However, the diabetic can also find cause for a lot of assurance. Much progress has occurred since Willis noted the sweet taste of urine in 1679. But it is a long way from Willis to Banting and Best to now. Since the development of insulin in

1921 and its use in humans later, progress has accelerated. Newer injectable insulins have been developed and insulin itself has been increasingly purified. The effect of the adrenals, pituitary and other glands on diabetes has been recognized. In 1955, the structure of insulin itself was determined. Immunoassays measuring circulating blood insulin have been developed. The use of the oral hypoglycemic agents in the mid-1950's stimulated interest in diabetes and at that time additional funds became available for the training of diabetologists. Insulin has been synthesized in several laboratories as early as 1960. More recently, proinsulin, glucagon, somatostatin and other substances discussed earlier have been defined.

This is only the beginning. The vision of diabetics is being aided by the proper use of laser beams. Limbs are being saved, whereas formerly whole wards of the New England Deaconess Hospital were occupied by patients who required amputations for complications of diabetes. Although amputations are still performed, modern surgical techniques have decreased the numbers markedly. Patients with defective kidneys are being helped with the use of artificial kidney machines and with transplants. Who knows what the future holds for the person with diabetes?

Just prior to the discovery of insulin, groups of young diabetics were kept virtual prisoners in metabolic wards. Such a group was housed in a cottage near the New England Deaconess Hospital. They were gaunt young men and women; the timely discovery of insulin gave them salvation. One of these patients was Dr. George R. Minot, who survived because of insulin and later won the Nobel Prize for discovering the treatment of pernicious anemia. Present-day diabetics are in some respects in the same situation. Although they no longer starve and they live useful lives, they too are living on the verge of great future developments from research.

the spirit of diabetes future

This Spirit would probably be the most exciting visitor for today's diabetic. The claim that little has been done for the diabetic is not valid. The problem is that so much has been accomplished that it is hard to organize the information and put it in proper perspective. The progress of research has changed from a trickle in 1920 to a torrent today. Small bits of research data can develop into meaningful progress. Consider this analogy: no one person really invented the automobile. Long ago the wheel was invented; then others discovered that if they put a frame and a box on the wheels, they had a wagon. This vehicle evolved, much later, into an automobile. Similarly, researchers have bits and parts that don't seem to fit anyplace, until eventually someone puts the pieces together into a very important finding.

Oral Insulin? A thought uppermost with many diabetics is the question, "Why can't I take insulin by mouth?" Insulin is a protein with two chains connecting a total of 51 amino acids. The body treats it as it would any other protein. The process of digestion separates the 51 amino acids so that they can be absorbed through the intestinal wall (no more than one or two amino acids can pass through the intestinal wall at one time). Insulin taken orally is absorbed, not as insulin, but as small bits and pieces, the 51 amino acids. Insulin has been synthesized on a number of occasions, but the process is extremely difficult and not economically feasible at present. However, the art of developing synthetics has been successful in many other areas, and it is probable that a practical method for synthesizing insulin on a large scale will be found some day, and possibly in a form that could be taken by mouth.

Pancreatic Transplants. Many diabetics have dreamed of the possibility of pancreatic transplants. However, this surgery is difficult to do. More than 50 such operations, in which all or most of a human pancreas was transplanted, have been performed in human subjects since 1966 specifically to improve the diabetes. A transplanted pancreas does function for a time, but unfortunately the rejection rate is high. To combat rejection, massive doses of immunosuppressive agents, including adrenal steroids, are required, and this increases the susceptibility to infection. Most transplants did not survive for more than a few months. Still, it was hoped that pancreatic transplants would improve the course of vascular disease in diabetes. However, at this time, pancreatic transplantation is not in the immediate future and it will probably never be a widespread remedy. Aside from the hazards of surgery and possible complications, diabetics who take daily injections of insulin survive reasonably well even without functioning beta cells of their own. Moreover, with eight million diabetics or more in the United States, where would the pancreases be obtained for transplantation?

Kidney Transplants. Kidney transplants have been much more successful and survival rates for diabetic persons given a kidney transplant have been as high as 65% for two years or longer. Vascular complications such as retinopathy seem to remain relatively stable after kidney transplantation. Many of these patients live reasonably normal lives.

Islet Cell Transplants. Islet cell transplants into similar laboratory animals have been extensively publicized. Although normalization of blood sugar is possible with such transplants in rats, rejection of the transplanted tissue has been a problem, unless the animals are inbred to make them genetically identical. Recently success has been achieved in transplanting beta cells from rats into culture media. The cells live and grow. When glucose is put in the culture media, the beta cells respond by releasing greater amounts of insulin. Cells from the culture which are transplanted into diabetic rats have been successful in that these animals have lived for periods of time without evidence of diabetes. The difficulty in moving this insulin-producing tissue from one species to another or even to animals of the same species is the formidable problem that has not been solved. Exciting progress has occurred, but further advances depend on improved research techniques yet unknown. When these difficulties are ultimately overcome, the technique may be considered for use in humans, but such is not the case now.

BETA CELL CAPILLARY TUBES. Because the host's body rejects transplanted beta cells, some researchers have devised a clever experimental method that uses bundles of thin capillary tubes enclosed by an outer chamber. Beta cells are placed in the outer chamber, around the tubes. Blood and nutrients can go through the thin capillary tube from intake and output openings, and they can penetrate the thin capillary tubes and bathe the beta cells. Insulin produced by the beta cells can also penetrate the thin tube walls and be carried away in the blood for use. However, the thin tube acts as a barrier filter that keeps the antibodies responsible for rejection away from the beta cells. This is an ingenious device that is an experimental procedure at present.

Artificial Pancreas. It is not difficult to get blood from a patient, take it to a computerized machine and get an accurate blood sugar measurement. Similarly, another computer could determine the insulin requirement and with the aid of a pump mechanism, inject the precise amount of needed insulin into the patient. If put into one large device and attached to a patient for a short period of time, this would be a completely computerized insulin-delivery system. There are several problems, however. These large, computerized, mechanical "pancreases" can be used only temporarily, since any direct connection with such mechanical units outside the body and the body's interior presents many hazards, including blood clotting and the possibility of infection, to say nothing of the size of the apparatus. However, it has been possible to build such a system and several are in operation (in Toronto, Canada, and Ulm, Germany, among other places). These units can be useful in hospital situations when, during an emergency, the patient could be attached to the apparatus for a period of time until the acute condition has subsided. However, such an apparatus is not feasible for everyday use. When this system is used, with a constant infusion of the ideal amount of insulin as needed, very little insulin is required, and the blood glucose level can be maintained close to normal.

The Glucose Sensor. The art of electronic miniaturization, learned during space exploration planning, has helped reduce the size of potential implantable electromechanical pancreases. These are under study in several centers. In some of these, it is not necessary to use only blood to determine the glucose content; body fluid bathing the cells can also be used. If a small sensor device, about the size of a quarter (*Fig. 36*) and suitable for implantation into subcutaneous tissue, is perfected, it might be used in a number of different ways.

A Glucose Monitor. It should be possible to attach to this sensor an appropriate miniature power supply and radio transmitter that would communicate with a small portable

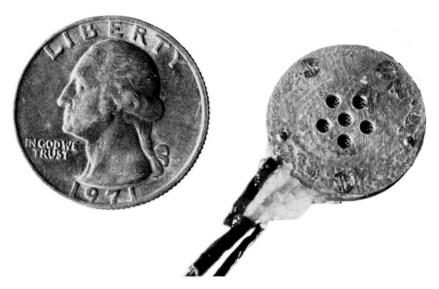

FIG. 36. A glucose sensor, compared in size to a quarter. This sensor could be implanted in subcutaneous tissue. (From Soeldner, J.S., et al.: Progress towards an implantable glucose sensor and an artificial beta cell. *In* Urquhard, J. and Yates, F.E.: Temporal Aspects of Therapeutics. New York, Plenum Publishing Corp., 1973.)

radio receiver designed to be carried conveniently by the diabetic. A transmission would take place every 15 minutes or so and be recorded by the receiver. The device could be constructed to set off an audible and/or a visual alarm if the glucose reading were lower than or exceeded preset levels. The patient could then anticipate a low blood sugar reaction or a period of excessively high glucose levels, day or night, and take appropriate prevention or treatment measures. This would be particularly useful in preventing problems with low blood sugar levels. A further refinement would allow the patient to plan insulin injections on a sounder basis than is now possible with urine testing. The content and timing of meals throughout the day could be changed to achieve better control of glucose levels. Newer gains in the development of miniature batteries (related to those used in cardiac pacemakers) would be usable in such a device. Eventually, a power package that could be recharged from external sources at weekly intervals will be developed. The patient could place a cloth-wire device over the area in which the "glucose monitor" was implanted inside the abdominal wall. This device would be attached to a suitable "black box" and from there to the household power source; after a night's sleep, the internal power unit would be recharged sufficiently for a prolonged period of use. The glucose monitor unit would be as small as half a pack of cigarettes; it would completely replace urine sugar measurement and make present-day blood glucose testing unnecessary in people wearing such a unit.

The Miniature Beta Cell. (Fig. 37)   If and when the preceding device is perfected, one more step would be needed to develop an artificial miniature beta cell; namely the addition of an insulin supply, pumps, computers and apparatus that would determine the insulin need and would provide the insulin required on demand. As projected, the system would

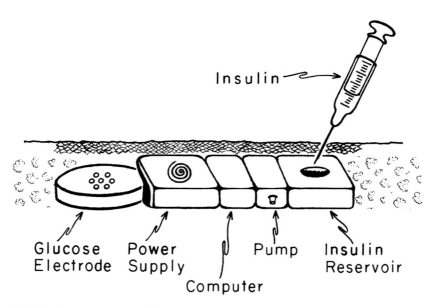

FIG. 37. A proposed model for an artificial miniature "beta cell," which would be implanted beneath the skin of the abdominal wall. The reservoir would be refilled with insulin by injection. (From Soeldner, J.S., et al.: Progress towards an implantable glucose sensor and an artificial beta cell. In Urquhart, J. and Yates, F.E.: Temporal Aspects of Therapeutics. New York, Plenum Publishing Corp., 1973.)

obviously require a reservoir for insulin, and since the whole device would be inside the abdominal wall, the insulin reservoir would have to be refilled by needle from the outside of the body. Regular (crystalline) rapid-acting insulin, in a higher concentration than currently available, might be needed. This goal is far from being reached at this time; it is hoped that the mechanical miniature devices might fill the gap until transplants of living cells becomes possible. Meanwhile, other methods yet unknown, such as the possible regeneration of flagging beta cells, might be perfected.

Other Research Hopes.   The role of other hormones and their influence on the diabetic state are being studied. For example, how do the beta cells recognize the concentration of blood glucose in the circulation? Receptors on the cell surface and their function are being investigated. Many substances can stimulate insulin release, including amino acids, which are the building blocks for protein.

Much has been learned about the processes causing a thickened basement membrane in the small blood vessels in the kidneys. Some investigators believe that early detection of this basement membrane thickening and earlier, more active treatment of diabetes can prevent later damage. At present, diabetes is often diagnosed *after* serious complications are found. A diagnostic marker that would detect diabetes earlier is needed. In any event, treatment probably should start much sooner.

Would an even purer type of insulin than now available be helpful to the patient? Would it result in less insulin resistance? One of the research hopes concerns a "beta cell cytotrophic agent," which could stimulate the pancreas to release more insulin right after the onset of diabetes. As mentioned previously, research into the influence of virus diseases on diabetes in young people is being conducted. Very little is known about the mechanism of the effect of diabetes on the large and small blood vessels, an area of vulnerability for the diabetic. What about genes? What is their influence? Can some type of genetic manipulation prevent diabetes?

These are only a few of the exciting possibilities that research might resolve in the future. But since the "Spirit of Diabetes Future" permits unlimited dreams, let's extend our imaginations even further into the dream world. As discussed in Chapter 1, all cells work by direction of a master set of plans called DNA, which is contained in the cell nucleus. This receives information regarding the environment of the cell, and if a particular protein is required, the DNA produces a "print-out" molecule called RNA, and then sends this messenger or transfer RNA to another area of the cell, where proteins are formed according to the plans derived from the DNA. Presumably, the cell could be directed to form any product, even insulin, depending on the messenger RNA. Suppose that in the future, we could give a proven harmless bacteria or a virus the messenger RNA with the information to permit insulin production. This organism might be injected into the patient. Could the bacteria or some virus then make insulin, or could the organism's message be used to stimulate the patient's beta cells, still alive but decreasing in function, to increase their output of insulin?

Another remote possibility is even more mind-boggling. Everyone develops from one cell, the fertilized egg. Yet, during development, each different cell knows exactly where to go and what to do. For example, the cells that form the liver, the heart and the pancreas all contain the same basic pattern of DNA, but somehow each has been programmed for different purposes and to perform different functions. The liver cell has been programmed to produce the enzymes needed for liver function; the beta cells are programmed to produce insulin. By determining the DNA pattern (gene) for producing a specific protein, such as insulin, perhaps in the future it may be possible to "reprogram" a liver cell, a skin cell, or any other body cell to produce insulin, thus making it work like a beta cell.

These are heady theories, far from realization, but as a pragmatic philosopher once said, "If you dream, dream first-class, it costs no more!" It is such dreams that stimulate researchers, who then go about making the discoveries that sometimes make dreams come true. After all, only a few years ago, most of the topics discussed in this chapter were unknown and sometimes undreamed of!

are attempts at control of diabetes worthwhile

Although there may be no complete uniformity of opinion on this subject, research and clinical advances during the past few years substantially support the belief that good control is vital. It is difficult to understand why anyone would espouse poor control. Physicians throughout the world strive constantly to achieve normality in every clinical and laboratory situation. Great efforts are made to keep temperature, blood pressure, blood electrolytes, urinary function, and every other function of the body within normal limits. It is difficult to understand why some people treat blood sugar levels in such a cavalier fashion. Can anyone be in favor of abnormality? True, the regulation of diabetes is extremely difficult in many diabetics, and indeed, it may even be necessary to purposely undertreat some patients to enable them to function. However, this is a choice dictated by necessity rather than a valid objective. At one time, medical authorities believed that modest elevations of blood pressure were not detrimental. Recent research has changed that attitude, and now authorities believe that "even a little bit is too much" as far as elevated blood pressure is concerned, although this attitude occurred after more effective blood pressure remedies were available. No one can deny that education and good control of diabetes can avoid acute complications. There is now some evidence that at least some of the long-term problems may also be postponed or prevented by better attempts at good diabetes treatment.

Some of this evidence is summarized in an official position paper prepared by three presidents of the American Diabetes Association and published in scientific journals, who stated that, "In the past few years, numerous studies in animals, including dogs, rats, monkeys, Chinese hamsters, mice, and others, have demonstrated that reduction of hyperglycemia by insulin therapy, by transplantation of insulin-producing tissue, or by other means, prevents or minimizes formation of diabetic-like lesions in eye, kidney, and nerve." The paper gives in some detail the reports that helped in the formation of these conclusions. The report further states that "these data therefore place the burden of proof upon those who maintain that diabetes control is without effect. The goal of appropriate therapy should thus include a serious effort to achieve levels of blood glucose as close to those in the nondiabetic as feasible." After pointing out that current means of treatment are not perfect and the development of more physiologic insulin delivery systems was important, the report concludes, "most important is a commitment to the view that better 'control,' when achievable, is beneficial."

Would anyone purposely choose inadequate control? The fact that the best available tools are imperfect should not deter one from the desire to build a good, solid house!

Results of Poor Regulation.   There has always been a strong clinical suspicion that poor regulation of diabetes helps to cause a higher incidence of complications. Certainly this proposition is unquestioned as far as the acute or short-term complications are concerned. The evidence is less firm about the long-term complications, about which the studies have often been retrospective (checking patient records afterwards, rather than by planned design in advance). Furthermore, it is difficult to find any significant number of patients who have maintained truly excellent control for any great length of time. More recently, pieces of the puzzle are being found that give more conclusive evidence. For one thing, the definition of the polyol pathway indicates that a continued high level of blood glucose causes accumulation of a degradation product called sorbitol in nerve tissue, in the lens of the eye and in other areas because normal metabolism is blocked. The accumulation of this undesirable substance may influence neuropathy and other degenerative results.

Excessive formation of other sugar-related products occurs with high blood sugar levels. These substances, "glycoproteins" in large amounts, may influence the thickening of the basement membrane of blood vessels in the eyes and kidneys, thus furthering deterioration. This effect is most noteworthy in the kidney. Examination of the blood vessels of the kidney with the high-power electron microscope has shown that, in diabetics, the membrane that lines the tiny vessels becomes thickened, causing, among other things, a loss of their ability to function as a filter. This filtering is one of the most important functions of the kidney. In studies with rats, it has been found that an enzyme involved in attaching sugars to the kidney membrane is more active in diabetic than in normal animals. This suggests that events leading to small vessel disease can be prevented and reversed by maintaining the blood glucose at normal or nearly normal levels.

For some time, evidence has shown that, along with poor control of diabetes, blood fat components such as cholesterol and triglycerides are often elevated. Recent studies also correlate undue elevation of blood glucose levels with a slowing down in the capacity of white cells to function, resulting in decreased resistance to infection. In any case the purpose of adequate treatment, whether by diet, the use of oral hypoglycemic tablets, or the use of insulin itself, is not simply to lower the blood glucose levels, although that is a byproduct. The goal is to have enough insulin available to permit the normal physiologic function of the body.

victory over diabetes

William F. Talbert, tennis champion, who has had diabetes for about 50 years since the age of ten, has said, "One must be the master . . . you or diabetes." Senator Gale McGee of Wyoming says, "Through the years we have discovered over and over that the greatest problem in diabetes is your state of mind." Mike Pyle, all-star center for the Chicago Bears football team, recalled that early in his diabetic career he used to feel sorry for himself. He overcame this with the thought, "I am not different from anyone else." He would often ask someone whether he appeared unusual. On being told he did not, he replied that he indeed was not sick—just a diabetic under excellent control. A whole book could be filled with such testimonials.

However, as important as are other persons' experiences, the final determination must be made by each individual. What it boils down to is that the person with diabetes must make a choice. He or she must accept the challenge of careful diabetic treatment or attempt to survive a career of carelessness. Obviously, patients need guidance at least periodically by physicians. No one can claim that the problem is simple or that by careful living with diabetes, all complications can automatically be avoided and a normal life span attained. There are still too many unknown factors, but good diabetes care pays dividends no matter how long the investment. Certainly the well-controlled diabetic feels better and is more useful and productive than the uncontrolled diabetic. People who continually fluctuate between elevated blood sugar levels verging on acidosis and continuous low blood sugar reactions are not completely effective.

In an earlier edition of this book, in a chapter entitled "Control of Diabetes and Why I Believe It Worthwhile," Dr. Elliott P. Joslin stated that there can be no argument that diet is extremely effective in treating the diabetic and that insulin in addition to diet can reverse the adverse effects of insulin deficiency. Dr. Joslin recognized that the diabetic life pattern was like a long race, and that people would succeed only if they were encouraged by running the race with others or by receiving some tangible recognition for their efforts. Thus, the awarding of various medals was instituted to provide this recognition.

The *Quarter Century Victory Medal* was intended to inspire patients to persevere in the careful control of their disease as well as to enable others to learn how they had achieved it. This medal was first given in 1948, to those able to document the fact that after 25 years of proven diabetes, they were in superb condition according to the following criteria:

1. Proof that diabetes has been present for 25 years (not always easy to document).
2. Certification by a physician that the patient's condition is generally excellent on physical examination and free from the complications usually considered due to diabetes. For example, the kidney function should be normal with no protein in the urine; the blood pressure should not be over 150/90.
3. Certification by an accredited ophthalmologist that the eyes are free from complications.
4. Certification by a radiologist that there is no evidence on X-ray films of any hardening or calcification in the arteries. X-ray studies usually include the chest, spine, pelvis, legs and ankles.

The *Life Expectancy Medal* has been awarded to more than 2000 patients. This is given to diabetics who have lived longer after the onset of diabetes than they would have been expected to live without diabetes. These criteria are based on

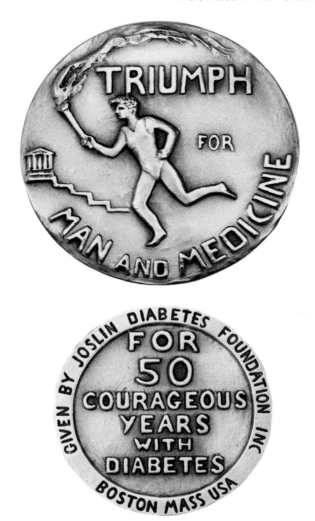

FIG. 38. The Fifty Year Duration of Diabetes medal. This medal is given to reward the courage and endurance of persons who have lived 50 years or longer since the onset of their diabetes.

life insurance tables prepared from the experience gained among persons in the general population.

The Fifty Year Medal (Fig. 38) is the latest and most important medal and is awarded to those patients who have had well-documented, insulin-requiring diabetes for 50 years or longer. No other qualifications are required. The depiction of the marathon runner on the medal is particularly significant in this award, because many of those patients who earn this medal contracted diabetes before the general use of insulin and, therefore, they had to live an unusually difficult and stringent life in the years before insulin. These persons are truly heroes. Nearly 200 of these medals have been given since 1970 to patients who, in most cases, have been extremely careful in their diabetes treatment. This number is growing constantly.

The achievement of a medal by a relatively few persons may not mean much in itself, except as a reward for those who have merited it. The important thing is that most of those patients who received these medals have been active people with great responsibility, who sometimes have lived more active and longer lives than their nondiabetic contemporaries. To live 50 years with diabetes means that the onset must have occurred at an early age for most of these victorious people. This should encourage many others. Such success can only be achieved by a person who is knowledgeable and motivated. He must also have the cooperation of his family physician and the love, interest and understanding of his family.

Dr. Charles H. Best, co-discoverer of insulin, has said, "Unfortunately, public knowledge of the advances in diabetes lags far behind the developments," and also, "Diabetics who take care of themselves have an excellent chance for a normal life."

It would be appropriate to close this first edition of the Manual written without the personal guidance of Dr. Elliott P. Joslin with an anecdote. Some years ago a young physician, while trying to examine a patient, was disturbed by the noisy and boisterous exertions of a young child patient. He was about to reprimand the youngster for his noisiness when the elder Dr. Joslin appeared and said, "Go ahead, son. Make all the noise you like." The young doctor, not understanding the intent of Dr. Joslin's words, could scarcely contain himself. However, Dr. Joslin continued by saying, "For many years we never saw or heard noisy children. They came here with diabetes and were very sick and very quiet. Often we did not see them again. It is exciting to see children well enough to behave like normal children." The young physician reflected and then decided that the noise really was not disturbing.

Only those patients and physicians who have lived through the periods before and since the discovery of insulin can realize how far the science and art of diabetes treatment have advanced in 50 years. At this point, research is on the verge of making many exciting and significant developments. Many diabetic patients will be alive to benefit from them. Already there is enough knowledge to enable people to live long, happy and useful lives. Many have. Many more are doing so. The best way to ensure the availability for the rewards of future scientific miracles is for diabetics to make full use of the knowledge and understanding of today.

13

What To Do Until You Can Reach Your Physician

Many minor emergencies worry persons with diabetes. Few of these are serious, but inexperienced diabetics and their relatives sometimes panic needlessly. When in doubt, call your physician, but if you cannot reach him, you can take certain measures. (All of these topics are discussed in more detail in the text.)

1. *How Do You Treat Diabetes During Acute Illnesses?*

Of course, diabetics, like those without diabetes, sometimes have illness that is not necessarily related to their diabetes, although many infections and acute illnesses make diabetes more difficult to treat. The "milder" diabetic who requires very little insulin or is treated with diet alone may not have a problem with control during sickness, but many diabetics suffering an infection of any severity may find the diabetes more unstable. At such a time, the patient often needs *more* insulin rather than less, in spite of the fact that the appetite may be poor, because insulin is usually less effective during illness. The urine tests for sugar must be checked much more frequently, and often supplemental doses of insulin are needed. At these times, urine specimens must be tested for acetone as well as for glucose. If acetone is present in any significant amount, contact the family physician at once (see page 104 and Appendix 7 for Sick-day Rules).

2. *How Do You Treat an Unconscious Patient?*

Unconsciousness may have many causes. Older persons may be subject to strokes and other cerebrovascular disorders. However, *if the onset is sudden* in patients being treated with insulin or oral hypoglycemic agents, one may usually presume that the cause is most likely hypoglycemia. While arranging for further medical care, it is safe to inject glucagon because other problems not involving low blood sugar will not be affected by this substance. (See page 152 for method of glucagon administration.)

3. *What Can You Do for Convulsions?*

These are usually self-limited. If the convulsion is due to low blood sugar, the patient should respond rapidly to the intravenous administration of glucose or sometimes to glucagon given subcutaneously. When the victim can drink, sweet liquids such as orange juice or ginger ale should be given.

In the event of a true epileptic seizure, put something between the victim's teeth to keep him from biting himself. A cloth wrapped around a stick is helpful; do not use your fingers. Generally these episodes pass quite rapidly.

4. *I Have Been Sick with the "Virus" and Can't Keep Anything Down. Since I Am Not Eating, Should I Eliminate My Insulin?*

No, not by any means! Insulin should be taken and the urine checked very carefully for sugar and acetone. Generally these acute episodes of nausea and vomiting do not last for any length of time; if not much is taken by mouth, the nausea often improves rapidly. When the acute nausea disappears, it is safe to start taking small amounts of bouillon, soup or even regular ginger ale, never taking more than a tablespoonful at a time until it is certain that the liquid can be kept down. Dry mouth and throat can be helped by sucking cracked ice, which melts and is swallowed gradually. If the urinary levels of sugar and acetone are significantly increased, consult the physician.

5. *Suppose I Find Acetone in My Urine?*

Urinary acetone can be found in many persons, especially in children on hot days, because they do not have enough available carbohydrate. It also occurs during fever but usually it is no threat unless it is accompanied by significant amounts of glucose in the urine. In that case, it may be a prelude to acidosis and should be treated with extra insulin, preferably under the direction of your physician.

6. *Suppose I Get a Sudden Blurring of My Vision?*

In the absence of any trauma or damage to the eye, the most common reason for temporarily blurred vision is low blood sugar. The treatment is to drink something sweet as soon as possible. Persons who are being treated vigorously, particularly with insulin, whose diabetes was previously uncontrolled, may have periods of blurred vision that are usually temporary and intermittent. These can be annoying and sometimes may last for several weeks (see page 153).

A marked loss of vision in a person known to have eye hemorrhages may represent an increased hemorrhage. If a person has increased hemorrhaging inside the eye, the best immediate treatment is to remain as quiet as possible and consult the physician as soon as possible.

7. *I Woke Up This Morning with a Wedge-Shaped Red Spot in the White of My Eye. What Is This?*

This usually is not related to diabetes and most often represents a subconjunctival hemorrhage due to irritation from rubbing the eye or some other cause. If not aggravated further, such spots tend to fade in several days.

8. *How Do You Treat Cuts and Bruises in a Diabetic?*

The same as in a nondiabetic. In case of bleeding, use pressure to stop the bleeding. Wash the area carefully with soap and water and apply a mild antiseptic such as ST-37. If the bleeding is severe or difficult to stop, medical attention will be necessary. Infection in persons who have well-controlled diabetes and good circulation is no greater a risk than in nondiabetic persons.

9. *I Have a Painless Black Toenail.*

If the dark area is limited to the toenail itself and there are no signs of inflammation or infection around the nail, it most often is due to hemorrhage beneath the nail caused by bruising the toe. Such an area usually fades and disappears after a few days or weeks. If the foot is painful, inflamed or discolored near or around the nail, the physician should be informed.

10. *What Should a Diabetic Do After Exposure to Poison Ivy, Poison Oak, or Poison Sumac?*

The same as anyone else. Wash the affected areas with large amounts of soap and water as soon as possible. In case of severe rash or eruption, see your physician.

11. *How Do You Treat a Sudden Insulin Reaction?*

Ordinarily, low-blood-sugar reactions are not a threat and are more often frightening and annoying than dangerous. However, too much insulin, too much activity, or not enough food intake can cause the blood glucose level to drop too low or too rapidly. At that point, symptoms may become severe enough that uncooperativeness, disorientation, or even unconsciousness develop. (This is discussed extensively on page 145.) Certain steps should be taken at once. Insulin reactions are nearly always preventable and when recognizeɑ, should be treated immediately. If a person is able to swallow, give the nearest available carbohydrate drink. Liquid is preferable to a solid because it is easier to swallow and is absorbed more quickly. Do not waste time looking for a particular drink such as orange juice if Coca Cola, ginger ale or any other sweetened liquid is nearby. Avoid calorie-free drinks at times like this; they are often used by mistake. If the person cannot swallow or does not respond, inject glucagon from a 1-mg. ampule and repeat with a second 1-mg. ampule shortly afterwards. If the patient still does not respond, take him to the nearest hospital emergency room for intravenous administration of glucose unless someone is available to give this injection at home. Insulin reactions that are short in duration or minor are not harmful, but they should not be permitted to become prolonged without treatment.

12. *It Is Now Noontime and I Forgot to Take My Insulin This Morning.*

This does not happen often. It is probably safest to take about two-thirds of the usual dose of intermediate insulin and add a few units of fast-acting regular insulin, supplementing with more regular insulin as needed at suppertime and bedtime according to urine tests. Better call your physician for guidance.

13. *I Took Too Much Insulin by Mistake. What Do I Do?*

If just a slight amount of excess insulin was taken inadvertently, no severe problem should develop, but sometimes people misread the insulin syringe and take twice as much insulin or more than they should. Don't panic. Simply take more carbohydrate or larger meals that day, supplementing these with orange juice or regular ginger ale and crackers between meals. It is better to eat and drink a little too much than too little at times like this. If too much nourishment has been taken, supplemental insulin can be used as necessary later. Small amounts of oral carbohydrate taken frequently are better than a single large meal.

14. *I Took Too Many Blood-Sugar-Lowering Pills (Oral Hypoglycemic Agents) by Mistake.*

Proceed the same as for insulin reaction, except that the action of blood-sugar-lowering tablets is usually more gradual and not as profound. However, in some cases the tablets may last longer, so precautions will have to be taken for a longer period.

15. What Do I Do if the Hypodermic Syringe and Needle Separate and Some Insulin Has Been Lost?

Try to estimate how much insulin remains in the syringe and how much might have been injected. If you are reasonably certain about how much has been lost, this can be replaced. If there is no way of determining how much has been lost, it is safest to check the urine before lunch, before supper and at bedtime and add further insulin as needed.

16. I Don't Remember Whether I Took My Insulin.

If doubt really exists about whether or not insulin was taken, carefully test the urine at intervals of several hours throughout the day, take small amounts of regular, fast-acting insulin, and consult your physician.

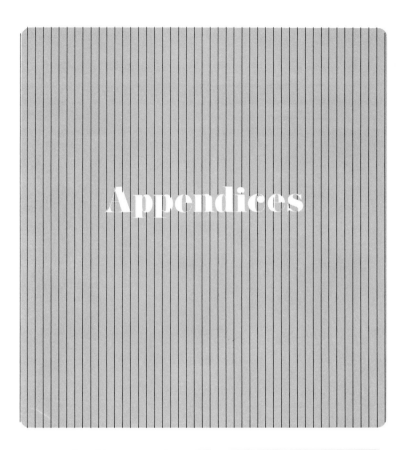

Appendices

appendix 1. useful addresses

The following organizations provide literature and information concerning diabetes:

JOSLIN DIABETES FOUNDATION, INC.
One Joslin Place
Boston, Mass. 02215

THE AMERICAN DIABETES ASSOCIATION
600 Fifth Avenue
New York, N.Y. 10020

JUVENILE DIABETES FOUNDATION
23 East 26 Street
New York, N.Y. 10010

INTERNATIONAL DIABETES FEDERATION
10, Queen Anne Street
London W1 M 0BD

ASSOCIATION FRANCAISE DE DIABETIQUES
5 ter, Rue d' Alesia
Paris (14'), France

BRITISH DIABETIC ASSOCIATION
10, Queen Anne Street
London W1 M 0BD

CANADIAN DIABETIC ASSOCIATION
1491 Yonge Street
Toronto, Ontario M4T 1Z5, Canada

For information concerning identification tags or bracelets;

Medic Alert Foundation
P.O. Box 1009
Turlock, California 95380

Much of the material included in the Appendices has been reproduced or adapted from *Diabetes Teaching Guide*, a publication of the Joslin Clinic Division of the Joslin Diabetes Foundation, Inc.

appendix 2. directions for following the diabetic diet

For every food category on the diet plan, e.g., meat, fruit, bread, there is a corresponding list from which you may choose an amount equal to that listed on your individual plan. Please review the rules for substitution if following a diet plan is unfamiliar to you.

Example: "Bread 1 slice" should refer you to the bread list. Everything on this list is equal in *food value* to 1 slice of bread. Therefore, you may substitute anything on this list anytime your diet plan says "Bread 1 slice." If you have "Bread 1 slice" for supper listed on your menu plan and you want potato: (1) use the bread list, (2) find "potato" (listed alphabetically), and (3) read across to the portion column (middle column), where it says ½ cup or ½ medium. That means that everytime you would like to have potato, you must eliminate 1 slice of bread and replace it with only ½ cup of potato.

If your plan says you may have "Bread 2 slices," that means you must use the equivalent to 2 substitutions. That is, 2 slices of bread equals 1 cup of potato with no bread or equals ½ cup of potato plus 1 slice of bread.

Example: Your menu plan also gives you meat portions. If your breakfast says "Meat 1 oz.," that means you must go the the meat list and choose whatever substitute you prefer for the meat, and then look to the portion column for the amount of that food to have, such as egg, 1 medium; peanut butter, 1 Tbsp.; or cottage cheese, 2 oz.

"Meat 2 oz." would equal double the portion of any substitute; "Meat 3 oz.," triple the portion.

All of the other lists are used in the same manner. Wherever a food is indicated on the menu plan, an amount equal to that may be selected from the corresponding list.

Three other lists require specific mention:

1. Small or Medium Fruit: Your diet will specify small fruit or medium fruit at different meals. Be sure to use the correct amount. Example: 1 small fruit = apricots ⅓ cup, while 1 medium fruit = apricots ½ cup.

2. "2 Uneedas" represents the standard for crackers and cookies (snacks). You may use any of the Uneeda substitutes from page 289 to replace your "2 Uneedas" in the snack. Example: "2 Uneedas" = Ritz crackers 5; or equals Saltines 4.

3. If your snack also includes milk, you may substitute the cracker part in the same manner as just explained and drink the $\frac{1}{2}$ cup milk or replace the entire snack. Example: "2 Uneedas plus $\frac{1}{2}$ cup milk" = 1 slice of bread plus 1 oz. meat with no milk. The bread and meat equals the crackers plus the milk.

FOOD SUBSTITUTIONS

Consistency is one of the important factors of the diabetic diet. Specific amounts of carbohydrates, proteins and fats should be eaten at certain times of the day, based on individual factors such as activity and insulin program. The TYPE of food consumed and WHEN it is eaten is as important as the total daily calories. This diet program is made more flexible on a daily basis by the use of substitutions, that is exchange of foods with similar values.

RULES FOR FOOD SUBSTITUTIONS

1. Substitute within the *same meal* or snack. Timing is important. If, for example, an egg will not be eaten at breakfast, some other protein source must be eaten AT THAT MEAL—not omitted and added to another meal.

2. Substitute *correct amounts.* In order to keep the food values of each meal consistent, it is necessary to know the correct amounts of each exchange. For example, 1 slice of bread (30 gm.) equals $\frac{1}{2}$ cup of cooked macaroni (75 gm.)

3. Substitute from the *same food family.* Each food family provides a different function for the body. For example, when quick energy is required, the body needs a carbohydrate rather than a protein food.

BREAD LIST

Each of the following is equivalent to bread, 1 slice (30 gm.), having the average *food value* of 15 gm. CHO and 2.5 gm. PRO.

FOOD	PORTION	WEIGHT
Bagel	$\frac{1}{2}$ average	30 gm.
Beans		
a. baked (without molasses & brown sugar)	$\frac{1}{4}$ cup	50 gm.
b. shell (lima, kidney, lentil)	$\frac{1}{3}$ cup	75 gm.

CHO = carbohydrate; PRO = protein.

BREAD LIST (Continued)

FOOD	PORTION	WEIGHT
Cereal		
a. dry	¾ cup	18 gm.
b. cooked	¾ cup	180 gm.
Chestnuts	5 large	35 gm.
Corn	½ cup	75 gm.
	(½ sm. ear)	
Corn bread	2″ square	45 gm.
Crackers	3 Uneeda Biscuits	See list
		page 289

(For further substitutes, multiply items in Snack (Uneeda) Lists by 1½ times each substitution. Ex.: 6 Saltines, 12 Wheat Thins)

Dry grated bread crumbs	¼ cup	20 gm.
Flour, tapioca, cornstarch,		
arrowroot	2½ Tbsp.	20 gm.
Fruit	medium	See list,
		page 288
Macaroni (Pasta)		
a. macaroni	½ cup	75 gm.
b. noodles	½ cup	75 gm.
c. shells	½ cup	75 gm.
d. spaghetti	½ cup	75 gm.
Matzo	one 6″ square	20 gm.
Melba toast	5 thin slices	20 gm.
Muffin		
a. bran	1 small	30 gm.
b. corn	1 small	30 gm.
c. English	½	30 gm.
d. plain	1 small	30 gm.
Parsnips	½ cup	100 gm.
Pilot Cracker	1	15 gm.
Popcorn	1½ cups	20 gm.
Potato	½ med.	75 gm.
	(½ cup whipped)	

CHO = carbohydrate; PRO = protein.

BREAD LIST (Continued)

FOOD	PORTION	WEIGHT
Rice	$\frac{1}{3}$ cup	75 gm.
Roll, dinner	1 small plain	30 gm.
Soup, plain vegetable type	$\frac{1}{2}$ can	100 gm.
	$1\frac{1}{2}$ cups (with water)	210 gm.
Sponge cake*	$1\frac{1}{2}$ in. cube	30 gm.
Squash, winter (baked)	$\frac{1}{2}$ cup	100 gm.
Sweet potato (yams)	$\frac{1}{2}$ sm. ($\frac{1}{4}$ cup)	50 gm.
Tomato sauce	$\frac{3}{4}$ cup	225 gm.
Water chestnuts	12	75 gm.
One hamburger roll	2 oz.	60 gm.
replaces bread	2 slices	60 gm.
One hot dog roll	$1\frac{1}{2}$ oz.	45 gm.
replaces bread	$1\frac{1}{2}$ slices	45 gm.

*To be used only for special occasions or for strenuous activity.

MEAT LIST

Each of the following may be substituted for meat, 1 oz. (30 gm.), having the average *food value* of 7 gm. PRO and 5 gm. FAT.

MEAT	PORTION	WEIGHT
Beef	1 oz.	30 gm.
Cheese	1 oz. (1 slice)	30 gm.
Cottage cheese	2 oz. ($\frac{1}{4}$ cup)	60 gm.
Egg	1 Medium	50 gm.
Fish	1 oz.	30 gm.
Ham	1 oz.	30 gm.
Lamb	1 oz.	30 gm.
Organ meats	1 oz.	30 gm.
Peanut butter	1 Tbsp. ($\frac{1}{2}$ oz.)	15 gm.
Pork	1 oz.	30 gm.
Poultry (fowl)	1 oz.	30 gm.
Shellfish		
a. clams, oysters, scallops, shrimp	5 small	30 gm.
b. butterfly shrimp, crab, lobster, etc.	1 oz.	30 gm.
Veal	1 oz.	20 gm.

CHO = carbohydrate; PRO = protein.

MEAT LIST (Continued)

MEAT	PORTION	WEIGHT

Meats that may be substituted occasionally if not on weight reduction diet or salt restricted diet:

Frankfurters	1 ($5\frac{1}{2}''$ x $\frac{3}{4}''$) or 3 (2" x $\frac{1}{2}''$)	50 gm.
Luncheon meat (cold cuts)	1 oz. (1 slice)	30 gm.
Sausage (pork)		
a. link	1	20 gm.
b. bulk	$\frac{2}{3}$	20 gm.

VEGETABLE LIST

A 1-cup serving (150 gm.) of a 3% vegetable is equal to a $\frac{1}{2}$ cup serving (75 gm.) of a 6% vegetable. Therefore, if your diet calls for 1 cup of 3% and $\frac{1}{2}$ cup of a 6%, you may instead have 2 cups of 3% or 1 cup of 6% if you prefer.

Example: Diet calls for 3% vegetable, 1 cup (150 gm.) + 6% vegetable, $\frac{1}{2}$ cup (75 gm.)

You may have one of the following choices:

1. String beans, 2 cups (300 gm.) and no 6% vegetable.
2. Tossed salad and broccoli, 1 cup (150 gm.) and no 6% vegetable.
3. Winter squash, 1 cup (150 gm.) and no 3% vegetable.

3% VEGETABLES: 1 cup (150 gm.) contains 5 gm. CHO and 2.5 gm. PRO.

asparagus	celery	kohl rabi	squash, summer
bamboo shoots	collard greens	lettuce	string beans
bean sprouts	cress, garden	mushrooms	swiss chard
beet greens	cucumber	mustard greens	turnip & greens
broccoli	dill pickles	radishes	water cress
cabbage	egg plant	rhubarb	wax beans
cabbage, Chinese	endive	sauerkraut	zucchini
cauliflower	green pepper	spinach	

6% VEGETABLES: $\frac{1}{2}$ cup (75 gm.) contains 5 gm. CHO and 1.25 gm. PRO.

artichoke	dandelions	onions	squash, winter
beets	green peas	parsley	(boiled)
brussel sprouts	kale	pimento	tomato
carrots	leeks	pumpkin	tomato sauce
chives	okra	red peppers	

CHO = carbohydrate; PRO = protein.

MILK AND MILK PRODUCTS

Milk is one food that contains a significant amount of all three food families: carbohydrate, protein, and fat. For example, 8 oz. (240 gm.) of whole milk could be substituted for bread, 1 slice (30 gm.), meat, 1 oz. (30 gm.), and butter, 1 tsp. (5 gm.).

If you use more than 3 oz. (90 gm.) of milk per day in coffee or tea, the additional milk must be included in your daily diet.

WHOLE MILK EQUIVALENTS

8 oz. whole milk contain 12 gm. CHO, 8 gm. PRO, 8 gm. FAT

Whole Milk	1 cup	8 oz.	240 gm.
Skim Milk + 2 tsp. butter	1 cup	8 oz.	240 gm.
Powdered Milk + 2 tsp. butter	$\frac{1}{4}$ cup	2 oz.	60 gm.
Buttermilk + 2 tsp. butter	1 cup	8 oz.	240 gm.
Evaporated Milk	$\frac{1}{2}$ cup	4 oz.	120 gm.
Yogurt (PLAIN ONLY) + 1 tsp. butter	1 cup	8 oz.	240 gm.

SMALL FRUIT LIST

Each of the following portions has an average *food value* of 10 gm. CHO.

FRUIT	PORTION	WEIGHT
Apricots	$\frac{1}{3}$ cup (3$\frac{1}{2}$ halves)	80 gm.
Apple	2$\frac{1}{2}$ oz. ($\frac{1}{2}$ med.)	70 gm.
Applesauce	$\frac{1}{3}$ cup	90 gm.
Banana	$\frac{1}{2}$ medium	50 gm.
Blackberries	$\frac{1}{3}$ cup	90 gm.
Blueberries	$\frac{1}{2}$ cup	70 gm.
Cantaloupe—Casaba	$\frac{1}{2}$ cup	150 gm.
Cherries	$\frac{1}{3}$ cup (13)	80 gm.
Cranberry juice (diet)	5$\frac{1}{2}$ oz.	160 gm.
Diet Cranapple Juice	1 cup	240 gm.

CHO = carbohydrate; PRO = protein.

SMALL FRUIT LIST (Continued)

FRUIT	PORTION	WEIGHT
Diet cranberry sauce	$\frac{1}{4}$ cup	120 gm.
Figs (fresh only)	1 large	60 gm.
Fruit cocktail	$\frac{1}{2}$ cup	100 gm.
Grapefruit	$\frac{1}{3}$ cup	100 gm.
Grapes	$\frac{1}{4}$ cup (15)	60 gm.
Honeydew melon	$\frac{1}{3}$ melon (5″ diam.)	130 gm.
Lemon	3 average	120 gm.
Mango	$\frac{1}{2}$ small	60 gm.
Orange	$\frac{1}{3}$ cup (1 small)	100 gm.
Papaya	$\frac{1}{4}$ medium	80 gm.
Peach	$\frac{1}{3}$ cup (2 halves)	100 gm.
Pear	$\frac{1}{2}$ cup (3 small halves)	90 gm.
Pineapple	$\frac{1}{3}$ cup (2 slices)	70 gm.
Plums	2 small	60 gm.
Prunes (cooked only)	3	50 gm.
Prune juice	$\frac{1}{4}$ cup (2 oz.)	50 gm.
Raspberries	$\frac{1}{2}$ cup	80 gm.
Strawberries	1 cup	150 gm.
Tangerine	1 large	90 gm.
Tomato juice	1 cup	240 gm.
Watermelon	1 cup	150 gm.

MEDIUM FRUIT LIST

Each of the following portions has an average *food value* of 15 gm. CHO.

Apricots	$\frac{1}{2}$ cup	120 gm.
Apple	4 oz. juice, 1 small	105 gm.
Applesauce	$\frac{1}{2}$ cup	135 gm.
Banana	$\frac{3}{4}$ medium	75 gm.
Blackberries	$\frac{1}{2}$ cup	135 gm.
Blueberries	$\frac{3}{4}$ cup	105 gm.
Cantaloupe—Casaba	$\frac{3}{4}$ cup	225 gm.
Cherries	$\frac{1}{2}$ cup	120 gm.
Cranberry juice (diet)	8 oz. (1 cup)	240 gm.
Diet Cranapple Juice	12 oz. (1$\frac{1}{2}$ cup)	360 gm.

CHO = carbohydrate; PRO = protein.

MEDIUM FRUIT LIST (Continued)

FRUIT	PORTION	WEIGHT
Diet cranberry sauce	⅓ cup	180 gm.
Figs (fresh only)	1½ large	90 gm.
Fruit cocktail	¾ cup	150 gm.
Grapefruit	½ cup	150 gm.
Grapes	⅓ cup	90 gm.
Honeydew melon	½ melon (5″ diam.)	195 gm.
Lemon	4½ average	180 gm.
Mango	¾ small	90 gm.
Orange	½ cup (1 medium)	150 gm.
Papaya	⅓ medium	120 gm.
Peach	½ cup (3 halves)	150 gm.
Pear	¾ cup (5 small halves)	135 gm.
Pineapple	½ cup (3 slices)	135 gm.
Plums	3 small	90 gm.
Prunes (cooked only)	4½	45 gm.
Prune juice	3 oz.	75 gm.
Raspberries	¾ cup	120 gm.
Strawberries	1½ cups	225 gm.
Tangerine	2 small	135 gm.
Tomato juice	1½ cups	360 gm.
Watermelon	1½ cups (chunks)	225 gm.

SNACK (UNEEDA) LISTS

Each of the following may be substituted for 2 Uneeda Biscuits plus ½ cup of whole milk, having the average *food value* of 16 gm. CHO, 6 gm. PRO, and 5 gm. FAT.

1. ½ cup cereal (12 gm. dry, 120 gm. cooked) plus ½ cup whole milk
2. 3 Uneedas plus 1 Tbsp. peanut butter or 1 oz. meat (no milk)
3. 1 medium fruit plus 1 oz. cheese
4. 2 Uneedas plus 1 tsp. butter plus ½ cup skim milk
5. 1 pkg. peanut butter Nabs (4 sandwiches) (no milk)
6. 2 Uneedas plus ½ cup D-Zerta pudding
7. 1 slice bread plus 1 oz. meat

Each of the following may be substituted for 2 Uneeda Biscuits, having the average *food value* of 10 gm. carbohydrate, 2 gm. protein, and 1 gm. fat.

SNACK (UNEEDA) LISTS (Continued)

FOOD	PORTION	WEIGHT
Animal crackers	6	
Arrowroot biscuits	3	
Brown Edge	2	
Butter Thins*	3	
Cheese Tidbits	20	17 gm.
Chocolate Snaps*	4	12 gm.
Ginger Snaps*	3	12 gm.
Graham Cracker	1 whole (2½″ x 5″)	14 gm.
Lemon Snaps*	3	11 gm.
Lorna Doones*	2	
Oyster Crackers	20	average 12 gm.
Pretzels (Nabisco Co.)		
Dutch	1	16 gm.
Pretzelettes	8	14 gm.
3-ring	4	12 gm.
Veri-thin	2	11 gm.
Veri-thin sticks	45	12 gm.
Ritz or Cheese Ritz	5	
Rye Thins	6	
Rye Krisp	2	12 gm.
Saltines	4 (2″ x 2″ each)	
Social Tea Biscuits	3	
Soup—Uncreamed	1 cup (with water)	150 gm.
Triangle Thins	10	
Triscuit	3	
Vanilla Wafers—small	4	
Vegetable Thins	8	
Waverly Wafers	4	
Wheat Thins	8	
Zwieback	2	
The AVERAGE	4 (½ oz.)	15 gm.
Bread	⅔ regular slice or 1 thin slice	20 gm.
Fruit	1 small	(see list, page 287)

*To be used only occasionally or for strenuous activity.
CHO = carbohydrate; PRO = protein.

BUTTER (FAT) LIST

Since butter and margarine are the same food value (fat) in equal portions (1 tsp., 1 pat), they may be substituted for one another. However, butter is derived from animal fat; margarine, from vegetable fat. This difference may determine which your doctor advises you to use.

Each of the following equals butter, 1 tsp. (5 gm.), average *food value* of 4 gm. FAT.

FOOD	PORTION	WEIGHT
Avocado	$\frac{1}{8}$ whole (4″ diam.)	25 gm.
Bacon	1 strip	7 gm.
Cream		
Heavy	2 tsp.	10 gm.
Light	1 Tbsp.	15 gm.
Sour	4 tsp.	20 gm.
Whipped	2 tsp.	10 gm.
Cream cheese*	2 tsp.	10 gm.
Salad dressing*	1 Tbsp.	15 gm.
(any regular commercial)		
Half and half	2 Tbsp.	30 gm.
Lard	1 tsp.	5 gm.
Margarine	1 tsp.	5 gm.
Mayonnaise	1 tsp.	5 gm.
Nuts		average 7 gm.

(Nuts also contain some carbohydrate and protein, which must be considered when taken in larger quantities than those listed below.)

Almonds	5	8 gm.
Brazil	1	6 gm.
Cashews	5	7 gm.
Filberts	4	6 gm.
Mixed nuts	5	7 gm.
Peanuts	11	10 gm.
Pecans	4 halves	5 gm.
Pistachio	15	7 gm.
Pumpkin seeds		6 gm.
Sunflower seeds		8 gm.
Walnuts	4 halves	6 gm.

CHO = carbohydrate; PRO = protein.

BUTTER (FAT) LIST (Continued)

FOOD	PORTION	WEIGHT
Oil		
Corn	1 tsp.	5 gm.
Olive	1 tsp.	5 gm.
Peanut	1 tsp.	5 gm.
Safflower	1 tsp.	5 gm.
Olives		
Black	2 Large	20 gm.
Green	6 medium	40 gm.
Peanut butter	1 tsp.	5 gm.

*When using the *diet forms* of these products, double the amount allowed on the meal plan, as they all contain ½ the calories of the regular forms.

MISCELLANEOUS SUBSTITUTIONS

FOOD	PORTION	WEIGHT	
Biscuit	1 small	35 gm.	Eliminate 1 slice bread plus 1 tsp. butter
Custard, baked, (artificially sweetened)	½ cup	120 gm.	Eliminate small fruit plus 1 oz. meat
Donut, plain	one medium (4″ diameter)	50 gm.	Eliminate 2 slices bread plus 2 tsp. butter
French Fries	10 small (½″ x ½″ x 2″)	50 gm.	Eliminate 1 slice bread plus 2 tsp. butter
Pancake*	1 average	45 gm.	Eliminate 1 slice bread plus ½ oz. meat
Pizza, plain cheese	3½ oz.	100 gm.	Eliminate 2 slices bread plus 1 oz. meat plus 1 tsp. butter
Potato Chips	1 oz. bag	30 gm.	Eliminate 1 slice bread plus 2 tsp. butter

*Do not use pancake-waffle mix. Use home recipe or pancake mix.

MISCELLANEOUS SUBSTITUTIONS (Continued)

FOOD	PORTION	WEIGHT	
Soup, creamed or chowder ⅓ can concentrate plus ½ cup milk	1 cup liquid	320 gm.	Eliminate 1 slice bread plus 1 oz. meat
Waffle	1 average	75 gm.	Eliminate 2 slices bread and 1 oz. meat
Wheat Germ	1 round Tbsp.	10 gm.	Eliminate ⅓ slice bread or 1 Uneeda biscuit or 6% vegetable ½ cup or 3% vegetable 1 cup
Wheat Germ	1 oz.	30 gm.	Eliminate 1 slice bread plus 1 oz. meat

30-GRAM FOOD CHART*
Carbohydrate, Protein and Fat in Basic Foods

	CHO	PRO	FAT
Bread, 1 slice	15	2.5	0
Uneedas, 2	10	1.5	1
3% Vegetables	1	0.5	0
6% Vegetables	2	0.5	0
Milk (whole)	1.5	1	1
Milk (skim or buttermilk)	1.5	1	0
Egg, 1 med. (50 gm. scrambled)	0	6	6
Meat, lean & fish (average value)	0	7	5
Chicken (all poultry & fowl)	0	8	3
Shellfish	0	6	0
Cheese, yellow	0	8	10

* Each food value is for 30 gms. (1 oz.) of that food unless otherwise indicated.
CHO = carbohydrate; PRO = protein.

30-GRAM FOOD CHART (Continued)

Carbohydrate, Protein and Fat in Basic Foods

	CHO	PRO	FAT
Cheese, cottage	0	4	1
Butter-5 gm., 1 tsp.	0	0	4

CEREALS

Cooked cereal, 180 gm.	15	2.5	1
Dry, prepared cereal, 18 gm.	15	2.5	1

FRUITS

Small list	10	0	0
Medium list	15	0	0

* Each of the food values listed is for 30 gms. (1 oz.) of the specific food unless otherwise indicated.
CHO = carbohydrate; PRO = protein.

LEARNING HOW TO CALCULATE YOUR DIET

Procedures for calculating: Divide the total weight of the food in grams by 30. Then multiply the result by the CHO, PRO, and FAT values given in the 30-gm. Food Chart for the specific food.

Example: What is the food value of 240 gm. (8 oz.) of whole milk?

Step 1. Find the food value for 30 gm. on Food Chart:
            Milk 30 gm. = 1.5 CHO, 1 PRO, 1 FAT

Step 2. Divide the total amount of milk (240 gm.) by 30 gm.:
            $240 \div 30 = 8$

Step 3. Multiply the amounts of CHO, PRO, and FAT in Step 1 by the answer in Step 2:

$$
\begin{array}{ccc}
1.5 \text{ CHO} & 1 \text{ PRO} & 1 \text{ FAT} \\
\times 8 & \times 8 & \times 8 \\
\hline
12 \text{ CHO} & 8 \text{ PRO} & 8 \text{ FAT}
\end{array}
$$

Therefore, 240 gm. of whole milk = 12 CHO, 8 PRO, and 8 FAT.

Using this procedure, calculate the food values of the sample portions listed in the chart on page 295.

FOOD	GRAM WEIGHT	CHO	PRO	FAT
Meat	120 gm.			
3% Vegetable	150 gm.			
6% Vegetable	75 gm.			
Butter	10 gm.			
Bread	30 gm.			
Milk	240 gm.			
Medium Fruit				

CHO = carbohydrate; PRO = protein.

FOOD LABELING

Recently it became law that all food manufacturers making a "claim" about their product, for example: "low calorie;" "new, improved," etc., had to list on the label of that product a breakdown of nutrients, including carbohydrates, protein and fat. This is done according to serving portions, which are often given in gram amounts. The total number of servings per container is also indicated.

This information is useful for persons with diabetes. Those who have learned how to calculate their diet in grams of carbohydrates, protein, and fat, versus those who use just the substitution lists in the book, are able to introduce a wide variety of brand name foods into their diet by using the information on the labels.

For example, if you have listed on your meal plan a snack of 2 Uneedas, you know from the Snack List that this contains 10 gm. CHO, 2 gm. PRO, and 1 gm. FAT. If you would like to use a brand of cracker that is not on the cracker list, but whose labeling indicates that each serving of 2 crackers = 6 gm. CHO, 1 gm. PRO, and 1 gm. FAT, you can determine how many Brand X crackers your diet plan permits, using the number that most closely approximates the food value of the 2 Uneedas:

$$2 \text{ Uneedas} = 10 \text{ gm. CHO}$$
$$2 \text{ Brand X crackers} = 6 \text{ gm. CHO}$$
$$3 \text{ Brand X crackers} = 9 \text{ gm. CHO}$$

In this case, you can eat 3 Brand X crackers.

This type of calculating may be done with a variety of foods and for any meal, if the principles of calculating a diet are understood, thereby allowing the use of more brand name foods. This canot be accomplished, however, when only ingredients are listed without regard to a particular serving size, as many products are.

SAMPLE DIABETIC DIET GUIDE

Name _____   Date: _____

Total Daily Diet: C.   P.   F.   Cal: Insulin

	Breakfast			Lunch			Supper	
				Alternate Meal Below				
	Portion	Gm.		Portion	Gm.		Portion	Gm.
Meat			Meat			Meat		
			3% Veg.			3% Veg.		
			6% Veg.			6% Veg.		
Bread			Bread			Bread		
Butter			Butter			Butter		
Milk			Milk			Milk		
Fruit			Fruit			Fruit		

WEIGH FOOD AFTER COOKING

Snacks: _____

  Forenoon   Afternoon   Bedtime

Alternate Meal

_____

_____

_____

appendix 3. dining out

APPETIZERS:

Order
1. Vegetable juices or unsweet-ened fruit juices.
2. Clear broths or bouillon, consomme
3. Fresh vegetables
4. Sour or dill pickles
5. Fresh fruit cup

Avoid
1. Canned fruits
2. Chowders
3. Vegetable or meat soups
4. Anything marinated in oil
5. Any meat or fish appetizers (unless amount allowed for main course is reduced)

SALADS:

Order
1. Fresh fruit or vegetable sal-ads without dressings (use lemon or vinegar)

Avoid
1. Salads with unknown dress-ings
2. Avocado (unless butter por-tion is reduced or elimi-nated)
3. Potato salad

VEGETABLES:

Order
1. Stewed
2. Boiled
3. Steamed

Avoid
1. Escalloped
2. Creamed
3. Au Gratin
4. Fried
5. Sauteed

POTATO:

Order
1. Mashed
2. Baked
3. Boiled
4. Steamed

Avoid
1. Creamed
2. Escalloped
3. Delmonico
4. Home fried
5. Browned
6. French fried (unless correct substitution known)
7. Potato salad

BREADS (WHITE OR DARK):

Order
1. Hard or soft rolls
2. Plain muffins
3. Biscuits
4. Crackers
5. Corn bread

Avoid
1. Sweet rolls
2. Coffee cake
3. Danish rolls
4. Frosted rolls

MEAT, FISH, OR CHICKEN (trim extra fat off):

Order	*Avoid*
1. Roasted	1. Fried
2. Baked	2. Grilled
3. Broiled	3. Sauteed
4. Boiled	4. Stewed
	5. Braised
	6. Breaded
	7. With gravy or bacon

EGGS:

Order
1. Soft
2. Hard
3. Poached
4. Scrambled ⎫
5. Fried   ⎬   Decrease Butter Allowance
6. Omelet   ⎭

FATS:

Order	*Avoid*
1. Butter	1. Gravy
2. Salad Dressing	2. Fried foods
3. Bacon	3. Foods with cream sauce
4. Cream	4. Salads with oils or dressing already mixed in them

DESSERTS:

Order	*Avoid*
1. Jell-O	1. Custards
2. Fresh fruit	2. Pies
3. Plain flavored ice cream	3. Sweetened canned fruits
4. Angel food cake	4. Pastry

BEVERAGES:

Order	*Avoid*
1. Sugar-free sodas	1. Postum
2. Coffee	2. Cocoa
3. Tea	3. Chocolate milk (or any flavored milk)
4. Buttermilk	4. Milk shakes
5. Whole milk	5. Regular soft drinks
6. Skim milk	6. Any beverage with unknown ingredients
7. Unsweetened fruit juices	

appendix 4. height and weight tables

Normal Height and Weight, Ages ½ to 21 Years

AGE	MALE		FEMALE	
	HEIGHT INCHES	WEIGHT POUNDS	HEIGHT INCHES	WEIGHT POUNDS
YEARS				
½	26	17	26	16
1	29	21	29	20
2	33	26	33	25
3	36	31	36	30
4	39	35	39	34
5	42	38	41	37
6	45	43	44	43
7	47	50	47	47
8	49	55	49	54
9	51	61	51	50
10	53	67	53	67
11	55	75	55	74
12	57	81	57	82
13	59	90	60	94
14	62	103	62	105
15	64	112	63	112
16	66	126	64	117
17	67	133	64	122
18	68	138	65	124
19	69	138	65	126
20	69	139	65	126

Desirable Weights for Men and Women
According to Height and Frame, Ages 25 and over

MEN

Height (In Shoes, 1-Inch Heels)		Weight in Pounds (In Indoor Clothing)		
FEET	INCHES	SMALL FRAME	MEDIUM FRAME	LARGE FRAME
5	2	112–120	118–129	126–141
5	3	115–123	121–133	129–144
5	4	118–126	124–136	132–148
5	5	121–129	127–139	135–152
5	6	124–133	130–143	138–156
5	7	128–137	134–147	142–161
5	8	132–141	138–152	147–166
5	9	136–145	142–156	151–170
5	10	140–150	146–160	155–174
5	11	144–154	150–165	159–179
6	0	148–158	154–170	163–184
6	1	152–162	158–175	168–189
6	2	156–167	162–180	173–194
6	3	160–171	167–185	178–199
6	4	164–175	172–190	182–204

WOMEN

Height (In Shoes, 2-Inch Heels)		Weight in Pounds (In Indoor Clothing)		
FEET	INCHES	SMALL FRAME	MEDIUM FRAME	LARGE FRAME
4	10	92– 98	96–107	104–119
4	11	96–101	98–110	106–122
5	0	96–104	101–113	109–125
5	1	99–107	104–116	112–128
5	2	102–110	107–119	115–131
5	3	105–113	110–122	118–134
5	4	108–116	113–126	121–138
5	5	111–119	116–130	125–142
5	6	114–123	120–135	129–146
5	7	118–127	124–139	133–150
5	8	122–131	128–143	137–154
5	9	126–135	132–147	141–158
5	10	130–140	136–151	145–163
5	11	134–144	140–155	149–168
6	0	138–148	144–159	153–173

appendix 5. dietetic foods

The diabetic patient should limit most foods labeled "dietetic." The word dietetic does not mean *diabetic* but applies to foods in which the caloric content or ingredients in general, and the carbohydrate content in particular, usually have been altered or decreased but not eliminated. The amount of alteration is often difficult to determine and the caloric content often remains high.

It is yet unproven that saccharin products used to sweeten many of the following dietetic items are harmful when taken in moderation. Excessive intake at one time of dietetic tonics, soda, candy, gum or jellies that contain a sweetner called sorbitol can result in positive urine tests for sugar and may cause diarrhea.

I. FREE ITEMS
  A. *Sugar substitutes*
     Label should state non-caloric or non-nutritive
  B. *Coffee additives*
     All powdered forms
  C. *Jams and jellies*
     1. Label should state: "5 calories per teaspoon" (or less)
     2. LIMIT: 1 teaspoon per meal
  D. *Soda or tonics* (dietetic)
     1. Label should state: "Sugar-Free"
     2. LIMIT: 1 quart per day
  E. *Gelatin desserts* (dietetic)
     1. Label should state: "Sugar Free"
     2. LIMIT: 3 half-cup servings per day
  F. *Diet candy*
     1. Label should state: 5 calories/piece (or less)
     2. LIMIT: 5 pieces/day

I. FREE ITEMS *continued*
  G. *Dietetic toppings:*
     1. Label should state: 5 calories/tablespoon (or less)
     2. LIMIT: 1 table-spoon/serving

II. DO NOT USE
  A. *Sugar substitutes*—
     Those *not* stating non-caloric or non-nutritive"
  B. *Dietetic cookies*, cakes, bread
  C. *Dietetic chocolate candy*
  D. *Dietetic sherbet, ice cream, custards, ice milk*
  E. *Coffee additives*, liquid or frozen forms
  F. *Instant breakfasts, breakfast bars, diet meals*

Show labels of foods in question to your physician, dietitian or teaching nurse for evaluation.

appendix 6. some commonly used insulins available in foreign countries

TYPE	COMMON NAMES
Short-acting (rapid)	
Clear, Crystalline, Regular	Usually identified by terms Actrapid, Insular, Insulina, Insulina Simple, Insuline, Insuline Simple, Insulyl, Iszilin, followed by manufacturer's name, such as Armour, Berna, Boots, Hoechst, Leo, Lilly, Novo, Organon, Roussel, Squibb, Welcome, and others.
Semilente	Made by a number of manufacturers; suffixes such as Demi-Dura, Semilente, Semilenta, and Sub-Tardum appear in name.
Intermediate (slow)	
NPH	Isophane, Rapitard, Retard, Protard
Lente	Suffixes such as Dura, Lenta, Lente, Lente Zinc, and Tardum appear after the name of the manufacturer.
Prolonged (very long)	
Protamine Zinc	Depotinsulin, Depot-insulyl, Depsulin, Endopancrine zinc-protamine, and Insulyl Retard are the commonest types. Nearly all are identified with the words "protamine zinc" in the name.
Ultralente	Often identified by Edtra-dura, Extra-Tardum or simply Ultra-Lente.

American made insulins are available in many countries; moreover, the new monocomponent (purest possible) insulins are available in the Actrapid, Semilente, and Monotard (intermediate duration) series in Europe.

appendix 7. sick day rules

Treat all illnesses as possible impending diabetic coma.

Sick Day Rules

1. Always take your usual daily dose of insulin. *Never omit it.*

2. Test your urine for sugar (Clinitest) a minimum of four times a day (i.e. before each meal and at bedtime).

3. Test your urine for ketones only if sugar is present. If you are too sick to test, someone must do it for you.

4. Rest, keep warm. Do not exercise.

5. Have someone at home to take care of you.

6. Take liquids every hour but do not force them if nausea and vomiting persist. Broth and clear soups can replace body salts lost in the urine. Record all food and liquid taken.

7. If in addition to feeling sick your urine sugar specimens are poor, you may need some extra insulin; *regular* (clear) insulin is used for this.

8. Although you are eating less than usual and are nauseated or vomiting, if your urine sugar specimens are poor (high sugar plus ketones), you *always* need additional insulin: *Regular* (clear).

9. *Ketones* in the urine are important *only* when sugar is also present and both are in large quantities. Under these conditions, the amount of insulin required may exceed the doses suggested, and you should seek help from your doctor.

NEVER give extra regular insulin if *only* the ketones are positive in the urine.

10. Although uncommon, diabetic acidosis and coma can develop in diabetic patients treated with diet alone or diet plus oral blood sugar lowering agent. During illness, these patients should also observe the sick day rules. At times, insulin treatment may need to be started under the direction of a physician.

11. Call your doctor for advice.

Regulation of Insulin on Sick Days

Take your usual dose of insulin.

Use regular insulin when supplementing your usual dose. Regular insulin looks clear in the bottle. It is important to have a vial of regular insulin on hand for emergency even if you do not use it normally.

Give extra insulin at specified times, preferably on the basis of second voided urine specimens.

Adding Regular Insulin on a Sick Day—Two Methods

The doses of insulin suggested here are subject to considerable variation. ASK YOUR OWN DOCTOR WHAT RULES HE WANTS YOU TO FOLLOW. However, one or the other method for supplementing the insulin dose is to be used *in addition to* the usual dose taken each day.

1. Units of Regular Insulin to be Added, *According to Age and Urine Test (Clinitest 5-Drop Method)*

	11:30 a.m.	*4:30 p.m.*	*Bedtime*
Adults			
If test is orange or brown*	12 U	12 U	12 U
If test is yellow	8 U	8 U	8 U
Children Under 10 Years			
If test is orange or brown*	6 U	6 U	6 U
If test is yellow	4 U	4 U	4 U
Children Under 5 years			
If test is orange or brown*	4 U	4 U	4 U
If test is yellow	2 U	2 U	2 U

*Rapid pass-through on Clinitest.

2. Adding 20% of the usual daily dose to the insulin dosage is a safe guideline for supplementing with regular insulin. The regular insulin may be given at three- to four-hour intervals or more often as directed by your physician.

Example:
1. Daily dose of 30 U NPH:
   20% of 30 U = 6 U regular insulin.
2. Daily dose of 10 U regular and 50 U NPH (60 U total):
   20% of 60 U = 12 U regular insulin.
3. Divided daily dose of 6 U regular and 24 U Lente before breakfast, and 10 U Lente at bedtime (40 U total):
   20% of 40 U = 8 U regular insulin.

Food Suggestions on Sick Days

			CARBO-HYDRATE	PROTEIN	FAT	CALORIES
Regular ginger ale	180 gm.	6 oz.	15	0	0	60
Regular cola drink	180 gm.	6 oz.	20	0	0	80
Grapefruit juice	150 gm.	5 oz.	10	0	0	40
Tomato juice	240 gm.	8 oz.	10	0	0	40
Cranberry juice	100 gm.	3.5 oz.	16	0	0	64
Hot cereal	120 gm.	½ cup	10	2.5	1	59
Milk	120 gm.	½ cup	6	4	4	76
					Total:	135
Egg Nog						
Combine						
Egg		1	0	6	6	78
Milk	180 gm.	6 oz.	9	6	6	114
Add						
Ice cream	50 gm.	¼ cup	15	2	8	140
					Total:	332
Dropped egg on toast (creamed)						
Egg		1	0	6	6	78
Creamed sauce-white	60 gm.	¼ cup	5	4	5	81
Bread	30 gm.	1 slice	15	2.5	0	70
Butter	5 gm.	1 tsp.	0	0	4	36
					Total:	265
Creamed soup	150 gm.	5 oz.	15	7	5	133
Saltines	10 gm.	4	10	2.5	1	59
					Total:	192
Scrambled egg	50 gm.	1	0	6	6	78
Butter	10 gm.	2 tsp.	0	0	8	72
Toast	30 gm.	1 slice	15	2.5	0	70
Milk	120 gm.	½ cup	6	4	4	76
					Total:	296
Creamed asparagus on toast						
Asparagus	150 gm.	1 cup	5	1	0	24
Creamed sauce-white	60 gm.	¼ cup	5	4	5	81
Toast	30 gm.	1 slice	15	2.5	0	70
Butter	5 gm.	1 tsp.	0	0	4	36
					Total:	211
Creamed asparagus on toast with bacon						
Bacon	15 gm.	2–3 strips	0	3.5	7.5	81.5
					Total:	292.5

Broth—Chicken, meat   FREELY

appendix 8. adjusting insulin doses

A. Guide to Adjusting Insulin Dose According to Blood and Urine Tests

INSULIN	TIME OF ADMINISTRATION	TIME OF BLOOD OR URINE SUGAR TEST (OR HYPOGLYCEMIC REACTIONS) AS BASIS FOR DOSE ADJUSTMENT			
		Before Breakfast	*Before noontime*	*Before Supper*	*Before Bedtime*
Regular	Before breakfast		X		
NPH or Lente	Before breakfast			X	
Regular	Before supper				X
NPH or Lente	Before supper	X			
NPH or Lente	Before bedtime	X			
Ultralente or PZI	Before breakfast	X (the following morning)			

B. General Notes

1. *The diet must be properly followed before considering any adjustment of insulin.*

2. Please refer to Table 7 for types of insulin, appearance, action, duration and peak of action.

3. At times of sickness, extra doses of regular insulin may be needed in addition to adjusting the daily insulin program. A sudden, dramatic change in the control of your diabetes (based on a change from the previous pattern of urine tests) may be secondary to sickness. See *Sick Day Rules,* Appendix 7, for further information.

4. Guidelines for insulin adjustment are rough estimates at best. There is obviously great variability among individual diabetic patients. Check with the physician who is responsible for the management of your diabetes to be sure he wants you to follow these rules. He may want to suggest a different schedule.

   Check with your physician if you are uncertain about how or when to adjust the insulin dose.

C. Adjusting Insulin Doses When Taking Morning Dose Only

   1. Guidelines for Increasing Dosage

      These guidelines should be followed only when the patient is in good health, but shows elevated urine glucose levels (the second-voided specimen tested by Clinitest method is yellow, orange or brown) for three consecutive days. *

      The dose of morning insulin is regulated by the result of the urine test done at the peak of action of the specific type of insulin. (See *Guide,* part A of this appendix.)

      a. If taking intermediate-acting insulin (NPH or Lente), increase dose by 2 units if the test before supper is poor for three consecutive days.

      b. Then, if the test *before lunch* is poor for three days, increase the *regular insulin* dose by 2 units the following morning.

      c. If taking *protamine zinc or Ultralente* insulin, increase dose by 2 units if the test *before breakfast* is poor for three days.

      NOTE: If the only consistently poor test is the pre-lunch test, always check with your own physician before increasing the dose of regular insulin more than once.

      Example: A patient routinely takes a mixture of 6 units regular and 20 units NPH insulin every morning. For three days in a row the pre-lunch test is poor, whereas the other tests are either negative or sporadically positive. The patient increases to 8 units regular and 20 units NPH without any apparent change in the test pattern. This patient should consult his physician before further increasing the dose of regular insulin.

   2. Guidelines for Decreasing Insulin

      Unless advised otherwise by your physician, decrease the insulin 2 units *only* for reaction, leaving the dose the same for blue tests.

      a. Before reducing the insulin dose for a reaction, always stop and try to think of some explanation for the reaction. For example: Was a meal late or was the amount of food consumed less than recommended in the diet? Was there a more than usual amount of exercise prior to the insulin reaction?

      If there is an explanation, do not decrease the insulin dose; rather, be more careful about adhering to the diet schedule or taking supplementary food to cover above-normal exercise.

      Remember, there is usually an explanation for insulin reac-

---

* Your physician may suggest increasing insulin when urine tests are poor for two consecutive days.

tions. If, however, no explanation for an insulin reaction can be found, then:

b. if the reaction occurs after breakfast but before lunch, decrease the regular insulin 2 units the next morning.

c. if reaction occurs at any other time of day, decrease the intermediate or long-lasting insulin 2 units the next morning. However, if this results in poor tests before breakfast, call your doctor at once.

d. *Do not omit* any dose of insulin without being told to do so by your doctor.

e. When the dosage has been changed, maintain the new dosage unless further adjustments are indicated by results of urine tests or by insulin reactions.

Exceptions to this rule:

a. Many patients with newly discovered diabetes enter a "remission phase" a few weeks after treatment with insulin is started and will require a rapid reduction in the insulin dosage. If you have newly discovered diabetes, be sure you have consulted with your physician and understand what a "remission" is and specifically how the insulin dosage should be adjusted during this phase.

b. Certain patients—typically juvenile onset diabetics whose disorder is of long duration—have diabetes that is difficult to control and tend to see a great deal of variability in their urine tests. This has been called *unstable* (or "brittle") diabetes. It is very unusual for such patients to have continuously negative (blue) urine tests for two or more days without also having insulin reactions, but if this does happen, the dose should be reduced by 2 units.

Caution: There are many patients who *think* or who have been told that they have unstable ("brittle") diabetes when this is really not the case.

Check with your own physician.

Do Not decrease your insulin dose for negative tests unless you have been specifically instructed to do so, or of course if you have symptoms of insulin reaction.

D. Adjusting Insulin Doses When Taking Morning and Bedtime NPH or Lente
   1. Guidelines for Increasing Dosage

      These guidelines should be followed only when the patient is in good health, but shows elevated urine glucose levels (the second-voided specimen tested by Clinitest method is yellow, orange or brown) for three consecutive days.

The doses of both morning and bedtime insulin are regulated by the result of the urine test done at the peak of action of the specific type of insulin. (See *Guide*, part A of this appendix.)
a. If the test *before supper* is poor for three days, increase the *morning NPH or Lente insulin* by 2 units on the next morning.
b. If the test *before lunch* is poor for three days, increase the *morning regular insulin* dose by 2 units on the next morning. See *Note*, part C of this appendix, for instructions regarding increases in regular insulin for *poor pre-lunch* tests.
c. If the test *before breakfast* is poor for three days, increase the *bedtime NPH or Lente insulin* by 2 units that night. (If both pre-breakfast and pre-supper tests are poor for three days, adjust the morning dose first.)

2. Guidelines for Decreasing Insulin

In general, guidelines for decreasing insulin for patients who take both morning and bedtime NPH or Lente are the same as for patients who take a single morning injection, with the exception of unexplained night-time insulin reactions.
a. If an unexplained insulin reaction occurs *before 2 a.m.*, it is probably due to the morning intermediate insulin, and this dose should be reduced by 2 units the next morning.
b. If an unexplained insulin reaction occurs *after 5 a.m.*, it is probably due to the bedtime intermediate insulin and this dose should be reduced by 2 units the next night.
c. Unexplained insulin reactions occurring *between the hours of 2 a.m. and 5 a.m.* can be secondary to the action of *either* the morning or bedtime intermediate insulin (or both). Consult your physician for his recommendation regarding which insulin dose to decrease.

appendix 9. oral hypoglycemic compounds, domestic and foreign brand names[a]

GENERIC NAMES	U.S. BRAND NAMES	FOREIGN BRAND NAMES	
Tolbutamide	Orinase	Artosin	Osdiabet
		Diabuton	Pramidex
		Dolipol	Rastinon
		Edudine	Sinadiabetes
		Mobenol	Tolbutone
		Orabet	Toluvan
		Oralin	
Chlorpropamide	Diabinese	Catanil	Diarinese
		Chlorodiabet	Melitase
		Chloronase	Mellinese
		Dabinese	P-607
		Diabetoral	
Acetohexamide	Dymelor	Dimelin	
		Dimelor	
		Ordimel	
Tolazamide	Tolinase	Diabewas	Tolinas
		Norglycin	Tolinese
		Orabeta	Tolisan
		Tolanase	
Glyburide	DiaBeta[b]	Daonil	Glibenese[c]
	Micronase[b]	Diaborale	Hemi-Daonil
		Euglucon	Maninil
		Euglocon	Minidab[c]
Phenformin[d]	DBI[d]	Asipol	Diabis Retardo[e]
	DBI-TD[d]	Biguanida	Dibein-Retard[e]
	Meltrol[d]	Retard[e]	Dibotin
		DB-Retard[e]	Dipar-Retard[e]
		DBI-Retard[e]	Glucopostin
		Debe-1	Glucopostin
		Debe-1-AP[e]	Retard[e]
		Debein	Insoral
		Debeone	Insoral AP[e]
		Debinyl	Insoral-TD[e]
		Diabis	

[a]Outside of U.S., combination of oral compounds within the same capsule are available (for example, tolbutamide and phenformin). These are not listed.
[b]Not yet approved for distribution in U.S.
[c]Actually glipizide, a chemical structure or formula similar to glyburide.
[d]Banned from general use in U.S. by the Food and Drug Administration.
[e]Indicates long-acting compounds.

appendix 10. urine testing materials

NAME OF TEST	MAKER	FACTOR MEASURED	TYPE OF MATERIALS	SCALE	COMMENTS
Clinitest, 2 & 5 Drop	Ames Co.	Sugar	Tablets, test tube, dropper and water	Colors differ for each % sugar—blue to orange, 0 to 2% or 0 to 5%	1. not specific for sugar 2. relatively bulky 3. moisture ruins tabs.
Clinistix	Ames Co.	Sugar	Strip test	Mauve, negative, to purple, positive	1. specific for sugar 2. same color shades often hard to distinguish 3. only measures to $\frac{1}{2}$% 4. timing important
Tes-Tape	Lilly	Sugar	Strip test	yellow, 0, to dk. green, $\frac{1}{2}$%, to dk. blue, 2%	1. specific for sugar 2. rapid 3. portable 4. moisture ruins tape
Acetest	Ames Co.	Acetone	Tablets and dropper	White, none, to deep purple, large amounts	1. rapid 2. timing important
Ketostix	Ames Co.	Acetone	Strip test	Buff, none, to deep purple, large amounts	1. rapid 2. easily portable
Diastix	Ames Co.	Sugar	Strip test	Color differs for each % sugar—light blue, to brown, 2%	1. specific for sugar 2. ketones may depress color development 3. rapid 4. easily portable
Keto-diastix	Ames Co.	A. Sugar B. Ketones	Strip test	A. As for Diastix B. As for Ketostix	A. As for Diastix B. As for Ketostix
Chem-strip G	Boehringer Mannheim	Sugar	Strip test	Yellow, 0, to pink, $\frac{1}{2}$%, to brown, 2%	1. convenient 2. result affected by large doses of vitamin C

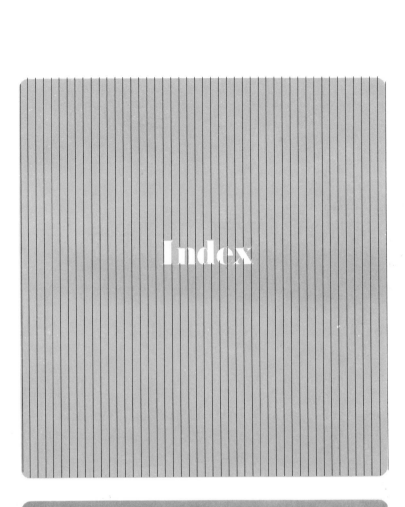

Index